DETACHMENT OF THE
RETINA

DETACHMENT OF THE RETINA

A CONTRIBUTION TO THE STUDY OF ITS CAUSATION AND TREATMENT

by

J. RINGLAND ANDERSON

M.C., M.B., B.S. (Melb.), F.R.C.S. (Edin.), F.C.S.A., D.O.M.S. (Lond.)

Ophthalmic Surgeon to the Alfred Hospital, Melbourne

WITH A FOREWORD BY

SIR JOHN HERBERT PARSONS

C.B.E., D.Sc., F.R.C.S., F.R.S.

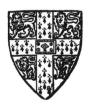

CAMBRIDGE

AT THE UNIVERSITY PRESS

Published for

The British Journal of Ophthalmology

1931

CAMBRIDGE
UNIVERSITY PRESS

University Printing House, Cambridge CB2 8BS, United Kingdom

Published in the United States of America by Cambridge University Press, New York

Cambridge University Press is part of the University of Cambridge.

It furthers the University's mission by disseminating knowledge in the pursuit of education, learning and research at the highest international levels of excellence.

www.cambridge.org
Information on this title: www.cambridge.org/9781107674981

First published 1931
First paperback edition 2013

A catalogue record for this publication is available from the British Library

ISBN 978-1-107-67498-1 Paperback

To

MY TEACHERS

SIR JOHN HERBERT PARSONS
&
J. HERBERT FISHER

CONTENTS

CHAPTER I

GENERAL

GENERAL. Definition. Retrospect. Aetiology. Influence of age, sex, occupation, heredity. The recognition of retinal detachment. The retina after detachment. The fundus after re-attachment. References

CHAPTER II

THE STRUCTURE AND FUNCTION OF INVOLVED TISSUES

The retina: its structure; its line of lowered resistance; its capillary system, permeability and pressure; its relation to the choroid; and its relation to the vitreous. The ora serrata. The choroid: its vascularity. The aqueous: origin and circulation. The maintenance of intra-ocular pressure. The vitreous: structure and optical effects. Turgescence and reaction. Turgescence and osmotic pressure. Reaction to injury and disease. References

CHAPTER III

PATHOGENESIS

THE THEORY OF DISTENSION. (*a*) Association of myopia. Pathology of myopia. Objections to this theory. Cystoid degeneration of the retina. (*b*) Association of trauma. Mechanism of trauma. Retinal tears. Frequency of tears. Macular holes. Traumatic macular holes. Spontaneous peripheral tears. Sudden detachment and retinal holes.

THE THEORY OF ATTRACTION. Leber's first theory: vitreous strands. Leber's second theory: preretinitis. Gonin's modification. Vitreous detachment. Criticism of traction theory.

THE THEORY OF DEPRESSION. The hydrostatic theory. The incidence of low tension. The causes of low tension. The effects of low tension. Detachment of the choroid. Hypotony in diabetic coma. Transudate or inflammatory exudate.

THE THEORY OF EXUDATION. Inter-retinal fluid. Inter-retinal haemorrhage. The influence of osmosis. Association with nephritis. Association with inflammation. Secondary retinitis. Association with sympathetic ophthalmitis. Influence of light and heat. Experimental work.

SUMMARY. References . . . .

CHAPTER IV

DIFFERENTIAL DIAGNOSIS

CHAPTER V

TREATMENT

CHAPTER VI

PROGNOSIS

APPENDIX

ILLUSTRATIONS

FOREWORD

THE vast increase of knowledge in every branch of science in recent times has of necessity impelled the division of labour to the extremes of specialism. Life is too short, even if mental capacity sufficed, to embrace all the accumulated facts of any one of the branches into which science has been conveniently, if unscientifically, divided. It is no longer possible even for the ophthalmologist to speak authoritatively on every aspect of his already restricted subject. One individual may efficiently write a student's manual or even a more comprehensive textbook; but the inquisitive searcher after detail will often find that he must have recourse to original papers in journals and the transactions of learned societies in order to satisfy his curiosity. Hence the need of larger encyclopaedias of composite authorship. More satisfying than these, however, are monographs, which gather together all the salient facts and theories of a sharply delimited universe of discourse and provide the research worker and others with a bibliography and critical apparatus, the foundations and sources of exhaustive knowledge.

Such a monograph is this by Dr Anderson on Detachment of the Retina. It embodies all the facts and theories relating to the subject, and discusses them with insight and good judgment, founded upon knowledge derived from patient research. It is only by a fortunate chance that empirical methods are successful in the treatment of a disease of unknown origin. It is only when the pathogenesis of the condition is understood that truly scientific treatment can be applied. Hitherto the pathogenesis of simple detachment of the retina has been to all intents and purposes unknown; and it must yet remain a subject of speculation until the physiology of the eye and its intraocular pressure has been further elucidated. The last few years have seen most encouraging signs of improved knowledge in this direction due to advances in biophysics and biochemistry. But there is a long road yet to traverse.

Meantime a ray of hope for sufferers from the disease under consideration has been afforded by a mode of treatment which is in its origin almost entirely empirical, but which fortunately in suitable cases is followed by an encouraging degree of success.

Dr Anderson's monograph is exhaustive and reliable. It is likely long to remain the chief source of information on Detachment of the Retina.

In conclusion I cannot refrain from expressing the hope that his example may be followed by many others who have time for laborious work of this nature; for such work confers a great boon upon their confrères.

J. HERBERT PARSONS

INTRODUCTION

CONSCIOUS of failure and yet encouraged by some slight success in the treatment of retinal detachment, the author has made an endeavour to study the literature. If the publication of his findings facilitates the approach of others to this subject, it will not have been in vain.

Though it is still too early finally to judge the merits of Professor Jules Gonin's theory and method of treatment, yet so many of his published results are triumphs compared with all previous ones that one anticipates a great step forward as a result of his brilliant and painstaking work. For this reason the present appeared an opportune time to make this publication.

The author has borrowed much from the published works of others, especially from the writings of Sir John Parsons, and from the Graefe-Saemisch-Hess Handbook. Of recent works, the many papers by Professor Alfred Vogt and Dr W. S. Duke-Elder have been of the greatest assistance. Anything of value in this book is solely due to such borrowings. It is hoped that easier access to views expressed in many journals and in diverse languages will be given through this book to those in busy practice. That the author is one of these is his excuse for the many deficiencies and the obvious defects in this publication.

I would like to place on record my gratitude to Sir John Parsons for his courtesy in honouring so small a contribution to ophthalmic literature by writing the Foreword to this book. Without his influence, and that of Mr J. Herbert Fisher, this book would not have been undertaken. To Miss McNab for skill and patience in typing, and to Miss Coverlid and Miss Gault for their help in translating lengthy German articles I am most grateful.

I must thank the Director of the Baker Institute, Dr W. J. Penfold, for providing the material necessary for experimental work, and Mr Edward Burt, a keen and efficient co-worker in any laboratory investigation.

Professor Vogt has been kind enough to permit me to reproduce some of his excellent illustrations. These are referred to in the text, and I am greatly beholden to him for his courtesy.

I must thank Dr T. àB. Travers for the help that he has given so willingly in the experimental work that initiated a thorough search of the literature, and in many other ways during the publication of this book.

J. R. A.

CHAPTER I

GENERAL: AETIOLOGY

GENERAL

DEFINITION. By Detachment of the Retina we mean a separation or cleavage of the two primitive retinal layers so that the pigmented epithelium remains adherent to the choroid, and the inner retinal strata of cells and fibres are separated from it. The retina is not completely detached, therefore this is an inaccurate title. It was the original title, and is universally adopted, therefore the continuation of its use appears to be desirable. Various pathological processes may account for detachment, such as an effusion of serum, blood, or pus, the growth of a tumour, the contraction of fibrous bands, the presence of a foreign body, or an entozoon.

With further investigation it is hoped that the terms "spontaneous" and "idiopathic" as applied to detachment of the retina will become less prominent. It is found that in many of these there is a history of trauma. In an eye predisposed to detachment of the retina by one of several different forms of degeneration, a surprisingly slight trauma can play the rôle of the exciting agent.

The importance of any detachment of the retina depends largely on the effect it will have on the total sight of the individual. It may be a mere incident of little value, as, e.g., in endophthalmitis. Here the underlying pathological basis is so potent as to destroy vision regardless of the additional retinal separation. Its importance however can hardly be overestimated when it results from a preretinal or subretinal haemorrhage which may clear up, leaving the detachment, or if when it occurs in the course of the degenerative changes in a myopic eye, the possibility of useful vision then depends on the end result of our treatment of the detachment. An understanding of the exact mechanism of its production is essential for successful treatment. No matter how overwhelming the causative lesion, it is wise to study and consider its effects, for only by so doing can one gain insight into the pathogenesis of detachment of the retina. On this depends the differential diagnosis and the success of treatment. Detachment due to such destructive disorders as Coats' disease, nephritis, sarcoma, etc., will be referred to and briefly discussed.

If one attempts to divide detachment of the retina into primary and secondary, it is only an artificial division based on the permanent effect and prominence of the underlying cause. If this is latent, the detachment appears to be primary, but if it is obvious and manifest, it is secondary. So all detachments of the retina will be considered as secondary lesions, and therefore as physical signs of some ocular or general disorder.

RETROSPECT. It is fitting before we proceed further to look back to the earliest recognition of detachment of the retina in the history of ophthalmology. The important books on morbid anatomy by Morgagni (1740) and de Krzowitz (1781) do not mention it. Earlier writers have mentioned animals' eyes in which it occurred, and the possibility of its occurrence in man. It is mentioned by St Yves (1722), but we find that he confuses it with "mouches volantes". It was not until much later that reliable histological observations were made by Ware (1805), Wardrop (1818) and Panizza (1826). It was called "hydrops subchoroidalis" to distinguish it from detachment of the choroid (hydrops subscleroticalis) which was in those days considered to be so much more common.

It was not seen *in situ* until expert observers like Chelius (1839), J. Sichel (1841), and Desmarres (1847) saw through the dilated pupil a white and at times vascularised membrane.

It was this appearance that Beer (1817) originally referred to as "amaurotic cat's eye". Invention of the ophthalmoscope was necessary before it could be studied clinically or any idea gained of its frequency. The first descriptions date back to Coccius, van Trigt, Arlt (1853) and A. von Graefe (1854). Certainly by his accurate clinical descriptions it appears that von Graefe fully proved the truth of the statement made by him, when first seeing the fundus with an ophthalmoscope, "Helmholtz has unfolded to us a new world". Because of their sudden onset von Graefe considered most detachments of the retina due to a subretinal haemorrhage. Stellwag (1856), as a result of his anatomical investigations, was able to disprove this idea. Arlt (1853) originated the theory of a choroidal effusion as the causative force, and five years later Müller showed that the organisation and contraction of connective tissue in the vitreous was the cause in certain eyes.

When Magnus (1883) was studying the various causes of complete blindness, he considered that 4·74 per cent. were due to retinal detachment. Evans (1929), when classifying 700 patients certified as blind, found retinal detachment in 4 per cent. and myopia the cause in approximately 3 per cent. More recently Cords (1930) has shown that myopia and bilateral detachment cause a higher percentage (19 per cent.) of blindness in the city of Cologne than any other disease.

AETIOLOGY

INFLUENCE OF AGE, SEX AND OCCUPATION. There are certain factors worthy of consideration. The first deals with the relation of age to the occurrence of detachment of the retina. Leber found that it was rare before the twentieth year, and that it gradually increased in frequency with increasing years. It appeared most frequent between the ages of fifty and sixty. Poncet (1887) and Walter (1884) found that about 66 per cent. of cases occurred after the age of forty. Stallard (1930) found 61 per cent. after this age. This preponderance becomes greater when we recall the obvious fact that there are considerably fewer patients alive after forty than before forty. Poncet (1897) found sixty to be the most affected age. Sattler (1905) found that males were more frequently affected than females; the proportion being 66 : 34. This disproportion is not due to the greater exposure of the male sex to injury, exclusion of non-traumatic cases from the statistics not affecting it. In Stallard's and Poncet's series, 62 per cent. were in males. Occupation does not appear to affect the incidence of retinal detachment. Magnus, who analysed a series of 243 patients, found that in half of them no special demands on the eyes were made. Leber and Poncet concurred with this view.

BILATERAL OCCURRENCE. The most marked variation occurs in the estimation of this point. Naturally if patients were followed over a longer period, and if detachments due to nephritis were included, a greater number of bilateral cases would be reported than in others which excluded these. Galezowski (1883) reported 9 per cent. of 551 patients and (1895) 2·5 per cent. of 1129. Deutschmann (1907), whose series included a very large proportion of severe cases, reported bilateral detachment in 32 per cent. of 220 patients. But Elschnig's figures (1914) are probably the most valuable. In 99 patients with non-traumatic detachment both eyes were affected in 25 per cent.

INFLUENCE OF HEREDITY. Treacher Collins (1892) and Clarke (1898) reported a family in which a brother and two sisters were affected. The condition was present in early life, and the parents were related by blood. In Arlt's family (1888), a woman, her son and granddaughter were affected. But here as in many other instances the patients were myopic, and it was this tendency that was inherited (Salzmann, 1921). In Kennon's family (1920), two brothers and one sister with otherwise normal eyes were found to have detachment of the retina. Previous injury excited the lesion in the males. Schreiber (1920) reported a mother and her son with bilateral detachment in non-myopic eyes. Pagenstecher's family (1913) was exceptional. Here the condition appeared to be transmitted from an affected male, through an unaffected female to two males. However, other ocular lesions were found in each patient as well. In three of the five members of a myopic family reported by Schmelzer (1929) a detachment was found. Pigmented areas in the retina and choroid of each affected eye were also seen. These were considered to be myopic in origin and the probable basis necessary for the detachment. Isolated cases associated with congenital coloboma of the iris and the choroid have been observed (Komoto, 1926; Wagener and Gipner, 1925).

CONGENITAL CASES. Numerous examples of retinal detachment found during the first few weeks of life have been reported. Some of these have been reported as pseudoglioma. In most cases foetal inflammation, with or without delayed involution of the hyaloid artery, appeared to be the most satisfactory explanation. Injury at birth explains some of these cases (Fernandez, 1905; Lachman, 1927; Marshall, 1897; Rockliffe, 1898; Fleischer, 1907). Onken (1928) has discussed the possible connection between naevus flammeus and retinal detachment.

THE RECOGNITION OF RETINAL DETACHMENT. The signs of an impending detachment are those due either to retinal irritation, choroidal inflammation, or some vitreous degeneration. Patients therefore frequently describe flashes of light, distortion of objects looked at, or an increasing number of black specks in the visual field. Once the separation has occurred, a cloud or a veil is often the way in which the field loss is described.

In Stallard's series (1930) a sudden onset is described in 52 per cent., and in 42 per cent. the onset was gradual.

Central vision need not be affected, even though a detachment has been present for many years. A patient reported by Lawson (1924), maintained 6/5 for at least fourteen months, even though there was a bilateral detachment present.

Two signs of interference with the rods and cones, or the visual purple, are an increase in light minimum and colourblindness for blue. This is a combination which is due either to congestion of the chorio-capillaris, or to some other upset in the functioning of the rods and cones. A loss of transparency of the fundus, a lack of brilliancy, and a very red fundus are further evidence of capillary congestion. Though at times green or blue vision is associated with retinal and choroidal diseases, coloured vision appears to be very rare in detachment of the retina. Beaumont found that the field for red demonstrated the extent of a tumour more accurately than the field for white.

The symptom which chiefly helps us in the recognition of a detachment of the retina is a loss of one area of the visual field, especially if the onset is sudden. The presence of myopia, the previous history of transient visual diminution, or the occurrence of some injury, are further evidence. Often the patient states that there has been for some time an appearance of flashing lights or sparks, or that objects looked at appeared distorted. Once the detachment is established, monocular diplopia may be found. The diagnosis is clinched if, through the pupil, either with or without the ophthalmo-scope, a greyish membrane is seen showing the characteristic ramification of retinal vessels. If, however, the media are not transparent, the difficulties of diagnosis may be great. The main signs then are reduced tension and a loss in the visual field. For a consideration of the difficulties in diagnosis see the section on "Differential Diagnosis".

As the pigmented layer of epithelium remains in contact with the choroid, the retina is at first transparent. Often when first seen it has become dull and grey, because it has been separated for some time from the choroid which nourishes so much of it. Later, as a result of atrophy, it becomes transparent again.

One characteristic appearance is the manner in which the vessels run over the undulating folds of the retina. They soon appear black in colour, because of the increased proportion of light reflected from the choroid. It is this dark appearance of the vessels and a tendency to tortuosity that gives one the greatest assistance in recognising a shallow detachment. The vessels later may show patchy infiltration of the lymph sheaths.

SLIT-LAMP FINDINGS. If an eye with a retinal detachment is studied with the slit-lamp one may find numerous dot-like deposits and well-defined and twisted fibres, due to coagulation of albumen in the vitreous. If myopia is present, the marked degeneration of the vitreous will be shown by the presence of prominent white fibres, narrow bands with transverse striation, fine white and brown dots and large masses which are fixed to the fibres and bands. Vogt (1921) finds a "dissolution" of the framework in high myopia. "Large areas appear optically empty, and on bulbar movement masses of fibre-like framework rapidly move." They do not gravitate, but usually return to their original location, so that we must presume that they are attached to a definite vitreous supporting structure—the "Glaskörperbasis" (Salzmann). Figure 353 in Vogt's atlas shows changes which he considered characteristic of detachment in myopia. Brownish red dots, evidently containing pigment, were attached to the framework, which itself in part was dissolved into fibres. The framework was more freely movable than usual and delicate white punctate changes and larger pigmented deposits were found. The retro-lental space was absent. If the tension is very low, the vitreous may assume a greyish yellow colour due to serous infiltration. When the retina has become atrophic its surface may show white masses or ramified lines over which run degenerate vessels ending in little coils. One may be able to discern dots of pigment epithelium adherent to its outer surface, and the subretinal exudate often appears stiff and of a dull yellow colour. A detachment due to inflammation with vitreous exudate may show numerous minute new vessels on the retinal surface and very delicate strands which radiate from its surface into the vitreous (Meesmann, 1927). Koby (1925) states that the vitreous framework is completely broken up in old myopic detachments. There are irregular and twisted fibres or large coloured platelets but no sign of a regular scaffolding.

THE RETINA AFTER DETACHMENT. The external layers of the retina normally receive their nourishment by osmosis, and it is possible that this process may continue even though they are separated from the pigment epithelium as in retinal detachment.

It appears that, even though the retina has been separated from its epithelial layer for some time, recovery of vision can occur. This is probably made possible by the filaments of the pigment cells growing in between the visual elements again. In an eye with typical detachment the retina was found only slightly raised from the choroid in two areas. The filaments were still present in a few places, but in most places they were broken off and formed a layer outside the rods and cones. As long as sufficient filaments remain intact, no changes in the rods and cones are noted, and vision may be as high as one-tenth with full perception of colour. If these connections are destroyed the rods and cones swell and become degenerate, the latter being more affected than the former. In old cases no trace of rods and cones may be found, and all the other cells appear degenerate (Speciale-Cirincione, 1925). The pigment epithelium shows an irregularity in the arrangement of its cells, and a tendency to proliferate through the subretinal space. The tendency for excrescences from the lamina vitrea (*drusen*) to form is marked. Areas of pigmentation and of fatty degeneration are found, and appear black, brown or yellow. White lines, due to cholesterin crystal formation, are further signs of degeneration. The yellow colour of the macula persists for a surprisingly long time after the development of a detachment (Vogt).

THE FUNDUS AFTER RE-ATTACHMENT. If a detachment has not been present too long, on re-attachment the fundus may assume its former appearance completely. As a rule, however, certain alterations are visible. These may be in the form of an irregular and dark pigmentation or a spotted appearance as in old choroiditis. This is due to the partial disappearance and the migration of pigment. But the most striking appearance is that described as "retinitis striata". The unsuitability of this term is obvious. It is wiser to adopt Schilling's classification (1903). He included under the title of "retinitis striata" any changes, due to inflammation, which assumed a striate arrangement; but the white lines following detachment he called "striae retinae". As far back as 1869, v. Jäger had recognised them and designated them "retinal cords".

After re-attachment one may observe these white retinal striae extending over a considerable area of the fundus (*v*. Plate 1). They are at times edged with pigment, and then may be raised, leading to undulation of the vessels which cross them. The striae are often about the same width as the larger retinal vessels. At times they branch. They lie deep

PLATE I

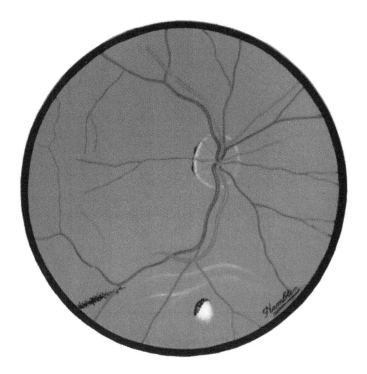

"Retinitis striata", and a healed hole. (Note that the vessels are
not deflected as they pass over the streaks.)

to the retinal vessels and the course of the latter is unde-
flected, or scarcely so at the intersections. This appearance
helps one to distinguish these strands from retinal folds
which cause considerable undulation of the vessels. Holden
(1895) suggested that striae may be due to the organisation of
subretinal haemorrhages. However, Fuchs considers that the
striae are generally, if not always, due to the re-attachment of
a detached retina. Leber (1877), Uhthoff (1894), Klainguti
(1923), and most histologists consider that the striae are due
to remnants of coagulated fibrin which take the place of the
neuro-epithelium, and which produce firm adhesions between
the retina and choroid. Slocum (1926) states that "the
peculiar streaks are probably choroidal exudates marking
the boundary of the detachment during stationary periods".
He considered that, as the subretinal fluid was absorbed,
new boundaries were formed, and that at these, striae of
coagulated exudation were left, like lines of débris which
mark the limits of the receding tide on the sands. In the
light of this evidence, there is little support for the theory
that this condition, known as retinitis striata, may represent
one of the causes of detachment (Lister, 1927).

REFERENCES

GENERAL

RETROSPECT

1722. St Yves. *Nouveau Traité des Maladies des Yeux*, 8, 331.
1740. Morgagni, J. B. *Epist. Anat.* 18, sect. 38.
1781. de Krzowitz, Tr. *Historia Amauroses*.
1805. Ware, J. *Chirurg. Observ. relat. to the Eye, etc.* 2nd edn., 1, 168.
1817. Beer, J. *Die Lehre von den Augenkrankheiten*, 2, 495.
1818. Wardrop, J. *Essays on the Morbid Anatomy of the Human Eye*, 2.
1826. Panizza. *Sul fungo midoll. dell' occhio*, Pavia. Deutsche Übers.
        Weimar, 1828.
1839. Chelius. *Handb. d. Augenheilk.* 2, 366.
1841. Sichel, J. *Ann. d'Ocul.* 5, 243.
1847. Desmarres. *Traité des Maladies des Yeux*, 1st edn.
1853. Coccius, A. *Über die Anwendung des Augenspiegels*, 125.
1853. van Trigt, A. C. *Der Augenspiegel und seine Anwendung*.

1853. v. ARLT, F. *Die Krankheiten des Auges*, 2, 158.
1854. VON GRAEFE, A. *Arch. f. Ophthal.* 1, 362.
1856. STELLWAG, C. *Die Ophthalmologie v. naturwiss. Standpunkt*, 2, 100.
1883. MAGNUS, H. *Die Blindheit, ihre.*
1929. EVANS, J. J. *Brit. Med. Jl.* 2, 847.
1930. CORDS, R. *Klin. Monatsbl. f. Augenheilk.* 84, 222.

AETIOLOGY

1883. GALEZOWSKI, X. *Recueil d'Ophtal.* 669 and 694.
1884. WALTER, E. *Klin. Studien über Netzhautablosung.*
1887. PONCET. *Bull. Soc. franç. d'Ophtal.* 5, 67; *Ann. d'Ocul.* 97, 236.
1888. v. ARLT, F. *Amer. Jl. of Ophthal.*
1892. COLLINS, E. TREACHER. *Ophthal. Hosp. Rep.* 13, part 3, 361.
1895. GALEZOWSKI, X. *Recueil d'Ophtal.* 385.
1897. BOURGEOIS. *Bull. Soc. franç d'Ophtal.* May 3, 368.
1897. MARSHALL, C. D. *Ophthal. Rev.* 397.
1898. CLARKE, E. *Trans. Ophthal. Soc. U.K.* 18, 136.
1898. ROCKLIFFE, W. C. *Ibid.* 18, 139.
1905. FERNANDEZ. *Arch. f. Ophthal.* 34, 338.
1905. SATTLER, H. *Deutsche med. Wochenschr.* 31, 1, 2.
1907. DEUTSCHMANN, R. *Deutschmann's Beitr.* Heft 67.
1907. FLEISCHER, J. *Verhandl. der Ges. deutscher Naturf.* 2, 288.
1913. PAGENSTECHER, H. E. *Arch. f. Ophthal.* 86, 457.
1914. ELSCHNIG, A. *Arch. f. Augenheilk.* 77, 2, 252.
1920. KENNON, R. B. *Virg. Med. Monthly*, July, 175.
1920. SCHREIBER, L. *Arch. f. Ophthal.* 103, 750.
1921. SALZMANN, M. *Wein. med. Wochenschr.* 24, 1082.
1925. WAGENER, H. P. and GIPNER, H. *Amer. Jl. of Ophthal.* 8, 694.
1926. KOMOTO, J. *Ibid.* 9, 414.
1927. LACHMAN, G. S. *Ibid.* Series 3, 10, 164.
1928. ONKEN, T. *Klin. Monatsbl. f. Augenheilk.* 80, 651.
1929. SCHMELZER, H. *Arch. f. Augenheilk.* 100–101, 268.
1930. STALLARD, H. B. *Brit. Jl. of Ophthal.* 14, 4.

THE RECOGNITION OF RETINAL DETACHMENT

1921. VOGT, A. *Atlas of Microscopy of the Living Eye*, Berlin. Trans. by von der Heydt, Plates 134, 353.
1924. LAWSON, Sir A. *Trans. Ophthal. Soc. U.K.* 44, 96.
1925. KOBY, F. E. *Slit-lamp Microscopy of the Living Eye.* Trans. by Goulden and Harris, London, 196.
1927. MEESMANN, W. A. *Atlas of Microscopy of the Living Eye*, Berlin, Plate 208.
1930. STALLARD, H. B. *Brit. Jl. of Ophthal.* 14, 1.

THE RETINA AFTER DETACHMENT

1925. SPECIALE-CIRINCIONE. *Ann. di Ottal.* 1925, **53**, 641.
VOGT, A. *Graefe-Saemisch Handb.* 3rd edn., Methods of Investigation, **3**, Plate 15.

THE FUNDUS AFTER RE-ATTACHMENT

1869. v. JÄGER, E. *Ophthalmosk. Handatlas* (fig. 73), 121.
1877. LEBER, TH. *Graefe-Saemisch Handbuch*, **1**, 5, 693.
1894. UHTHOFF, W. *Berliner kl. Wochenschr.* **37**,
1895. HOLDEN, W. *Arch. f. Augenheilk.* **31**, 287.
1923. KLAINGUTI, R. *Zeitschr. f. Augenheilk.* **50**, 71.
1926. SLOCUM, G. *Contrib. to Ophthal. Science*, 210. Edward Jackson vol., Wisconsin.
1927. LISTER, Sir W. T. *Brit. Med. Jl.* (Dec.), 1127.

CHAPTER II

THE STRUCTURE AND FUNCTION OF INVOLVED TISSUES

It is wise to emphasise the structure of certain tissues, which assume special importance when one considers the various mechanisms suggested to explain retinal detachment. One must recall the inherent weaknesses of such structures as well as their vital functions.

THE RETINA: *its structure*. The retina is a delicate transparent inelastic membrane. It extends from the optic disc to a point 4 mm. from the ciliary processes, where it ends in a dentated margin known as the ora serrata. Developmentally it is divided into two primary layers, the pigmented retinal epithelium, which represents the outer wall of the primary optic vesicle, and the whole of the remaining tissue which forms the inner wall. This tissue is composed of alternating layers of nerve cells and connecting fibres, and a framework of supporting fibres and neuroglia. There are three layers of cells and three of fibres, and together they represent three neurones on the path of the transmission of visual impulses to the brain. The main supporting structure is that formed by Müller's fibres, the end plates of which unite to form the external and internal limiting membranes. The outermost cell layer is divided into two parts by the external limiting membrane. This is a very delicate membrane, perforated like a sieve. Through its openings pass the cells of this layer which are the cells of the rods and cones. The outer projections of these cells form the rods and cones, and the inner nucleated extremities are superimposed, and the layer so formed is known as the outer nuclear layer. These cells constitute the first neurone. The main difference between the rods and the cones is in shape and size. At the fovea the cones become longer and more slender and resemble rods, but, in common with cones elsewhere, they do not contain obvious visual purple. The cells of the rods and cones form a mosaic, which, being represented accurately in the projected field of vision enables separation of visual impressions into their component details. The outer granular layer is one which varies greatly in different animals. As there is a granule for each visual element, and as those corresponding to the rods are five times as thick as the elements themselves, it follows that, for economy in space, the cells must be superimposed in several rows. The more numerous the layers, the finer and more numerous will be the corresponding rods and cones. The thickness of this layer may be considered as an index of the number of rods present, whether it be in different places in one retina or in the eyes of different animals. It is thickest in fish and mammals.

The inner nuclear or granular layer is very complicated, containing a variety of cells. The majority of the granules are the nuclei of the cells of the second neurone—the bipolar cells. The other cells present are the horizontal and the amacrin cells. The nuclei of Müller's fibres are also found in this layer (Greef, 1900). Few capillaries pass beyond the limits of this layer, and consequently morbid conditions with a vascular basis are most frequently found here.

The thickness of the retina varies in different parts. The variations are worth recalling. Near the optic nerve Kollicker found the retina to be 0·22 mm. thick; near the posterior pole 0·135 mm. (Krause 0·164 mm.), at the equator 0·084 mm. (Krause); and at its anterior margin 0·09 mm. The marked thinness of the ganglion-cell and nerve-fibre layers helps to explain this increase in delicacy towards the ora serrata. The ganglion cells are eight to ten deep in the yellow spot, and near the periphery they cease to form even a continuous layer. Towards the outer limit of the retina the nerve-fibre layer is only 0·004 mm., but near the entrance of the optic nerve it is 0·2 mm. in thickness. On the temporal margin of the papilla it is only one-half as thick as on the other margins, and it grows thinner still as the fovea is approached. This is significant in the consideration of retinal tears and their prevalence towards the periphery and the fovea. Ida Mann (1928) has shown that there is practically no increase in the thickness of the retina after the 21 mm.

stage. Any growth is in area only. This is in striking contrast with the growth of the other derivative of the fore-brain, the cerebral vesicle. Further, it can be shown that apart from morbid changes the retina shows no structural change after puberty. Probably even the identical cells persist from this time on throughout life. Not only does the width of the retina lessen towards the periphery, but so also does that of the choroid and the sclera does likewise. The sclera is approximately 1 mm. at the posterior pole, and an average width for the choroid is 0·25 mm. But near the equator each is thinner by 50 per cent.

The early appearance of Müller's fibres (10 mm. stage) enables them to form a scaffolding for the building of the more highly specialised tissue. They form the framework of the retina throughout life, and according to Cajal (1893) play an insulating part. Their innermost extremities, the footplates, unite to form the membrana limitans interna. Ida Mann has shown an apparent direct continuity between these fibres and the early vitreous fibrils. They appear to play a large part in the production of the primary vitreous. This and the subsequent formation of the vitreous from the optic cup helps us to understand the separation of this membrane from the retina which occurs clinically in a subhyaloid haemorrhage. Though in excised eyes the vitreous is not widely adherent to the retina the relationship during life is probably much more intimate.

THE RETINA: *its line of lowered resistance*. The invagination of the primary optic vesicle which begins at the 4·5 mm. stage is due to its own inherent power. The outgrowing retina, by the cytoclesis it exerts, calls the cornea and the lens into being (Wood-Jones and Porteous, 1929). The invagination leads to the formation of two layers, which later come into contact but do not unite. It is this line of contact which becomes a line of cleavage in the development of a retinal separation or detachment. This line appears to be a developmental "weak spot" or a line of lowered resistance. Until the end of the third month of foetal life the intervening space is ciliated, just as are the corresponding cavities within the brain and spinal cord. When the embryo is very small (10 mm.) two changes occur in the outer wall of the optic cup. Pigment granules appear and the cilia disappear from its inner surface. The cilia on the opposing surface of the inner wall probably increase in size as they diminish in number, and form the primitive outer limbs of the rods and cones. The latter lie within the cavity of the primary optic vesicle and early appear to adhere to the pigment epithelium. This attachment throws light on the adherence of these two layers when the mature retina becomes separated or detached by artificial or morbid conditions. It is wise to consider the cells of the rods and cones, viz. the neuro-epithelium and the pigmented epithelium, as a unit, anatomically, physiologically and pathologically. When the pigmented epithelium degenerates after choroidal disease, the neuro-epithelium is also affected and the pigment migrates. This migration and the ability of the lamina vitrea to proliferate probably aids the re-attachment of the retina when it is re-applied. It is remarkable that "there is no increase in thickness of the epithelial layer during this stage (*i.e.* up to 10 mm.), or indeed throughout life, it remains always only one cell thick as it was at its first appearance" (Ida Mann, 1928).

There is little in the criticism of the human retina by certain anatomists on the ground that it is "inverted" with the sensitive elements lying posterior to the several layers of cells and fibres. One must remember the transparence in ordinary light of the retinal nerve fibres when non-medullated. A striking contrast is shown by the opacity of these fibres when examined by red-free light, a quality that makes this light of such value. One must also remember that, as a result of the posterior position of these elements, they lie close to the rich network of choroidal capillaries. A rich network of such vessels before the retina, even though in the form of a pecten, would very seriously interfere with the transmission of light. The high product of evolution—the foveolar cones—are not covered by any layer and are protected by a yellow pigment. In this region there are no retinal vessels. The area is surrounded merely by a wreath of terminal capillary branches.

In passing it is well to recall the fact that the transparence of the media, the retina and even that of the retinal vessel walls, does not develop, but that it is the original embryonic state. The remaining tissues which are opaque during post-natal life were once transparent.

THE RETINA: *its capillary system, permeability and pressure.* The vascularisation of the retina is similar to that of the central nervous system. It is a vascularisation from the surface. On the outer surface there is the chorio-capillaris, and on the inner surface the retinal system which sends fine branches into the retinal tissue (Spalteholz, 1923). The former nourishes the rods and cones which constitute the functioning unit of the retina, the latter supplies the con-ducting apparatus—the various cells and their nerve fibres. It is interesting to note here the close resemblance in structure during the fourth month of foetal development between the retina and the cerebral cortex (Ida Mann).

Round even the smallest branches of the arteries and veins there is a characteristic perivascular sheath. These sheaths surround spaces which are connected with a network forming a definite system of lymph spaces (Koeppe, 1918). Salzmann has found the vessel walls poorly developed, especially the muscular wall of the arteries. Increased permeability may produce oedema, not only of inflammatory but also of non-inflammatory origin, as in contusions, and according to Fuchs, in Oguchi's disease, where the grey macular appearance is known as Mizou's phenomenon. A greater permeability may lead to the formation of a haemorrhage. From Friedenwald's investigations (1924–5) there appear to be two distinct net-works of retinal capillaries. The more superficial network lies in the nerve-fibre layer. The vessels tend to run parallel to the nerve fibres with short connecting branches crossing them. The deeper layer is only connected with this by widely separated channels. It lies mainly in the inner nuclear layer, but sends occasional loops down toward the nuclei of the rods and cones and upwards to the ganglion cell layer (Frieden-wald, 1924–5). "It may be stated as an axiom that the functional activity of every organ of the body depends upon

the rate at which blood circulates through its capillaries"
(Maitland Ramsay, 1929).

Krogh (1922) and more recent observers have shown that
normally the capillaries are relatively impermeable to colloids, but that light and heat rays and the influence of toxins,
poisons and drugs can increase the permeability so that
larger molecules can pass through. When there is an alteration in the blood content of diffusible substances (such as
sugar and chlorides) there will be a corresponding change in
the concentration of the intra-ocular fluids. An alteration in
the colloid content of the blood will scarcely influence the
number of the larger molecules which enter the aqueous,
unless the permeability of the capillaries is increased. That
this is possible has been shown by Krogh and others. It
occurs at death after the sudden lowering of intra-ocular
pressure; during inflammation, as one of the effects of toxins
and poisons, and as part of the reaction to heat, light, drugs,
or any other irritant or stimulus that would either dilate the
capillaries, or damage their walls.

It is too early to realise the influence that the new teaching
concerning capillary circulation will have on ocular problems.
For no longer is the state of the capillaries to be considered
a fixed one, but rather that they form "the most active,
purposive and dynamic part of the vascular system. All
vital processes take place through their walls" (Bryson,
1924). In considering capillary pressure it must be remembered that it is constantly changing, and that the range of
variation is wide. Apart from other evidence the high
pressure of intra-ocular tissues, viz. 25 mm. Hg compared
with 1–2 mm. elsewhere, is sufficient proof of normal high
capillary pressure in the eye. The rich ciliary network of
capillaries is capable of such wide distension that ten cor-
puscles can pass through it at a time, instead of in single
file as elsewhere (Fusita, 1919). This and the constricted
exits of the veins as they pass out of the eye are further
evidence of high capillary pressure.

When one observes the clouding of the media and ocular
tissues on excising an eye, one realises the vital part played by
the capillaries in maintaining ocular tension, and the high

degree of transparency that is so essential. A loss of translucency of the walls of a vessel is an early sign of disorder.

THE RETINA: *its relation to the choroid.* The pigmented
epithelium of the retina consists of a single layer of hexagonal
cells. The pigment appears brown over the choroid and
black when anterior to the ora serrata. A nucleus lies in the
unpigmented portion nearest to the choroid. The more
remote portion contains numerous pigment granules. The
number of these granules varies with the individual, being
very sparse or actually absent in albinism. Because this
layer remains attached to the choroid when the retina is
stripped off it was once considered part of it. The chorio-
capillaris "appears *pari passu* with the pigment" and is in
some way related to it. If for some reason the one does not
develop the other will be found absent. Which exerts the
determining influence is not known.

Just as the chorio-capillaris is richest behind the fovea,
so the retinal epithelial cells are smaller (12 instead 16–18
microns), more densely packed, and more deeply pigmented
here than elsewhere. This produces the darker colour of the
central area of the fundus. The protoplasmic filaments also
protrude more deeply between the cones than elsewhere.
Fortin (1930) believes that the delicate extremities of the rods
and cones establish the connection with the pigment epithelium. He does not consider that rods and cones are of unequal
length, but that the extremities of the cones are very fine, and
long enough to reach the choroid. As they are very fragile,
they are broken in ordinary sections and appear short. In
Halben's opinion (1910) the union between these two layers
is much firmer than is usually supposed.

Though it has not been conclusively proved that the visual
purple is secreted by the pigmented epithelium as Kuhne
suggested, these epithelial cells may yet have protective and
optical functions. The inner surface of the ciliary body and of
the iris is rough, but the choroid presents a smooth surface,
and it has been deduced that the choroid reflects light on
to the rods and cones. In Kepler's opinion, the choroid
absorbs light and does not reflect it. The cells of the pigmented

epithelium send in minute cilia-like processes between the rods and cones. Not only do the cones contract under the influence of light, but there is also an increase in the length of these cilia and a migration of pigment granules along them. In certain animals the completed light-position is assumed in about ten minutes, but it takes more than an hour for the typical dark position to be assumed (Arey, 1926). This may be a means of protecting the visual elements from intense light. It certainly explains why the retina clings more tenaciously to the choroid when the eye has been illuminated (Boll). It is of value to compare with this the findings in Oguchi's disease. The white-grey colour of the fundus is due to the migration of the pigment in the retinal epithelium on exposure to light. This pigment is more abundant and more active than usual, and Oguchi considers it atavistic (Oguchi, 1925–6). Sakai (1920) found in one patient with Oguchi's disease that on shading one-half of an eye the fundus appeared normal whilst the exposed half showed the typical pigment migration. Little is known of the influence of drugs on the retinal epithelium, but that such may appear clinically is shown by the disappearance of this epithelium in both eyes of a patient given too large an intravenous dose of an iodine preparation septoiod (Scheerer, 1926). A greyish oedema of the retina appeared followed by pigmentation and the development of a "pepper and salt" fundus. Similar changes can appear as a result of the influence of toxins liberated in such an infection as typhoid fever (Fuchs, 1930). There is considerable evidence to show that these cells and the visual purple are affected by bile and some of its salts. Rats treated with these showed degenerative changes of the pigment epithelium and night-blindness (Sugita, 1926). This throws light on the clinical association of jaundice and night-blindness in man. The value of liver-feeding in hemeralopia or hesperanopia is an established fact. This treatment has been recommended as well in early retinitis pigmentosa (Trantas, 1929). It is not known whether the liver actually forms visual purple or a hormone which enables the pigmented epithelium to secrete it, but the diminution in its formation in liver diseases, biliary obstruction and certain blood diseases is beyond doubt. As these conditions may be permanent there is the possibility of the development of fundus changes similar to those in retinitis pigmentosa. This form of retinitis hepatica is not likely to develop if the cause is transient. The hesperanopia in scurvy epidemics (28 per cent., Poskrowsky, 1924), pregnancy, anaemia, lack of food, especially of fats (Oguchi, 1919), and of vitamins, alcoholism (Lundsgaard, 1924), after excessive glare from snow, etc., in association with retinal and choroidal disease is probably due to deficient formation or to destruction of visual purple or the retinal epithelium.

Frequently one observes migration of retinal pigment in morbid conditions. It is seen most typically in retinitis pigmentosa, advanced myopia, various forms of choroiditis, and following contusion. After degeneration of the rods and cones the pigment appears free to migrate through the openings left in the external limiting membrane.

THE RETINA: *its relation to the vitreous.* For a long time there has been uncertainty regarding the existence of a hyaloid membrane. It has been held that two membranes existed between the retina and the vitreous, viz. the membrana limitans interna, and the hyaloid membrane. At present the majority of anatomists consider that only one membrane exists and that is, the anatomically demonstrable "glass" membrane lying inside the basal cones of Müller's fibres, known as the membrana limitans interna retinae. It continues over the fovea without interruption, but is lost round the entrance of the optic nerve and at the ora serrata.

The membrana limitans interna is most intimately connected with underlying retinal structures at the macula. This explains the well-known superficial folds which radiate from this point in the form of a macular star. This is modified in papilloedema and appears as a fan, because of the attachment of the retina to the disc and the block in circulation at this point. The direction of retinal folds is determined by the points of retinal fixation. The adherence of this membrane at the macula is further demonstrated by the maintenance of its light reflex in an early central subhyaloid haemorrhage. After a time it may disappear, but at first it is clear, and a briskly moving arched reflex may run from it over the curving slope of this membrane's surface.

Salzmann (1907) and Iwanoff have described a proliferation of Müller's fibres into the vitreous. This shows the possibility of a defect in the dividing membrane, and a union between the retina and the vitreous that is clarified by the facts known about the development of the primary vitreous.

The vitreous is fixed to the disc and less firmly to the inner surface of the retina. It is attached most firmly to the ora serrata and to the adjacent zone, 1·5 mm. broad, of ciliary epithelium. When the vitreous shrinks during hardening or fixation, or under pathological conditions, it clings to this area. If a severe injury does tear it free, the ciliary epithelium goes with it. This adherent part of the vitreous is known as the base of the vitreous. Salzmann (1912) describes a posterior and an anterior border-layer of the vitreous. It is simply the rind or condensed outer layer. The posterior border-layer extends from the base posteriorly along the retina. It dwindles as it reaches the posterior pole, but it is sufficiently adherent to the membrana limitans interna, near the optic disc, to remain so when the vitreous is detached. This border-layer is adherent to the membrana limitans interna retinae throughout. The anterior border-layer runs from the base anteriorly. It is separated from the analogous membrana limitans interna ciliaris by the posterior chamber, except in the posterior zone. Here fine vitreous fibrillae are attached to the orbiculus ciliaris and they intertwine with the posterior fibres of the zonule of Zinn.

THE ORA SERRATA. This is the well-defined, macroscopically perceptible serrated extremity of the pars optica retinae. It separates the retina from its very thin extension over the ciliary region known as the pars ciliaris retinae. The teeth of this serrated or toothed border correspond in position to the intervals between the ciliary processes. Methods of value in the examination of this area are referred to in the chapter on differential diagnosis. It is sufficient here to quote Egger (1924). "The ora serrata region is often to be recognised as a zone of meridionally placed parallel palisades which are not infrequently separated by pigment. These palisades also show the direction of the zonular fibres which spring from this area."

The retinal vessels become sparse and are not found within one millimetre of the actual retinal border, neither are ganglion cells nor nerve fibres found in this narrow zone. Of the visual cells the rods are the first to vanish, the cones which continue becoming simpler in form. Of the other layers the inner reticular layer is the last to disappear. The radial fibres of Müller, which form the main part of the supporting structure, persist and are highly developed. Just as there is this developmental displacement of the ora serrata backwards there may be a forward movement in certain conditions of disease. Fuchs describes this as an occasional result of extensive leucoma or marked staphyloma of the cornea. These changes produce a strain on the suspensory ligament of the lens and so on the retina. This explains the anterior position of the periphery of the retina. The gliding forwards of the retina on the choroid leads to degeneration of the retinal cells with gliosis and migration of pigment and the formation of changes resembling those characteristic of retinitis pigmentosa. Donders (1877) found that the extreme periphery of the retina was blind, a fact difficult to understand, for, even though the other cells are absent, the rods and cones extend to the very border. If, however, as Salzmann states, the rods in a zone 3-4 mm. wide at the periphery are devoid of visual purple, this is more easily understood. More recently the periphery has been found blind to green only (Ferree and Rand, 1920).

Not only is the ora serrata a transitional zone, but it is also an area of growth. Though during life the whole eye increases in volume 3·29 times, yet almost certainly the only division of cells taking place in the retina occurs in the region of the ora serrata (Ida Mann). At birth this area and the fovea are more foetal in character than the remainder of the retina. At the seventh month of foetal life it is level with the middle of the ciliary muscle, by the ninth month with its posterior border, and at term behind it. After birth the ora continues to move posteriorly. As the retinal border moves

backwards the teeth of the ora serrata become more prominent, and narrow radial striae—the striae ciliares—are seen
to run across the orbiculus ciliaris. To each tooth of the ora
serrata there is a corresponding stria lying in the valley
between the corresponding ciliary processes. Not only is the
distance of the ora serrata behind the ciliary muscle an
indication of individual age, but also of evolutionary advance;
a narrow ciliary region being common in the lower mammals.

The zone anterior to the ora serrata for a distance of four
millimetres is smooth and darker than the retina. It is known
as the orbiculus ciliaris or the pars plana of the ciliary body.
In it the retina is represented by a single layer of the slender
columnar cells which originate from the blended inner and
outer granular layers. The outer surface of these cells is
joined to the extension of the pigmented retinal epithelium
known as the pigmented epithelium of the ciliary body. As
this union is considerably firmer than that between the
choroid and the retinal pigment epithelium artificial detachments stop at the ora serrata. On the inner surface there is a
well-defined membrane, the limitans interna ciliaris. It tends,
like the limitans interna retinae, to disappear towards the
ora serrata (Salzmann). The intimate adherence of the pars
ciliaris retinae to the vitreous is a finding of importance.

The attachments of the ora serrata are worthy of summary:
Anteriorly the retina is continued on as the pars ciliaris and
the pars iridica retinae, and so attachment to the iris is made.
The vitreous is adherent at the ora serrata on the inner
surface, and externally the pigmented epithelium is adherent.
The suspensory ligament of the lens is attached by bundles of
fibrils to the pars ciliaris as far back as the ora serrata. These
fibrils are attached at those places which correspond to the
intervals between each pair of ciliary processes. The ciliary
processes unite the ciliary body to the choroid and so indirectly to the retina. This gives an indirect attachment to
the "tensor of the choroid", which is the outermost part of
the ciliary muscle. It is inserted into the choroid about mid-
way between the equator and the ora serrata. Brücke, who
discovered this muscle, considered that it stretched the
choroid and the retina over the vitreous, but Donders con-

sidered its attachment to the choroid a fixed point, and that it pulled the base of the iris and the inner wall of Schlemm's canal backwards. It is probable that both these actions occur (Gullstrand). The influence that accommodation may have on the retina because of these attachments is demonstrated by the "accommodation phosphene" (Helmholtz, 1924).

Not only is the region of the ora serrata the part of the retina most exposed to tension, but it has the disadvantage of being supplied and drained by the distal extremity of a vascular system. The vessel net gradually increases in simplicity towards the ora. "The loops have a somewhat wider calibre than the rest of the capillaries, and if one so wishes, one may speak of a direct transition of arteries into veins here" (Salzmann). Ebbecke in his entoptic experiments (1920) found that this part of the retinal circulation was the first to be affected by pressure applied to the eye and that with increasing pressure the periphery of the field was the first to fail. The ora serrata is also the area in which extension occurs late in embryonic life, and it probably shares the inherent weaknesses characteristic of other transitional zones.

It is of interest to note that the ora serrata and the fovea are similar in several respects. They are zones of transition which retain their foetal characteristics longer than other areas. They alter considerably during the first few years of life. The retinal vessels and the nerve-fibre layer are most sparse here. These areas are most susceptible to the development of cystoid degeneration.

It is well to notice the presence of three potential spaces. The perichoroidal, the inter-retinal and the pre-retinal or subhyaloid spaces. The first is crossed by several nerves and vessels and delicate lamellae. When the choroid is detached these bonds of union, especially the vortex veins, limit the spread of an effusion and aid absorption. An effusion into either of the other two spaces is influenced by gravity and changes its position accordingly. In each case re-attachment is first found in the upper part of the detachment.

Some light is thrown on the age-incidence of retinal detachment, when we recall the following changes which come with the passage of years. Not only does the sclera become more rigid, but the connective tissue increases greatly in the choroid, and in the bases of the ciliary processes. There is also a tendency for the pigment epithelium to atrophy and for colloid excrescences to form on the lamina vitrea. Kerschbaumer (1888, 1892) describes a loss of transparency and a thickening of the choroidal vessels as a frequent finding after the third decade of life. These changes and the cystoid degeneration to be discussed later must be kept in mind when considering the pathogenesis of retinal detachment.

THE CHOROID: *its vascularity*. The most striking feature about the choroid (the chorioid) is its vascularity which resembles in richness that of the chorion around the embryo. This richness suggests the nourishment of some vital tissue. Vital indeed, for let the well-being of the cones suffer, and all the maintenance of intra-ocular tension, the delicate balance of physical and chemical forces, and the transparence to and the accurate refraction of light, are in vain. Then too, not only the nine months of slow development of the individual, but also the age-long evolution of the type would have been rendered almost futile.

The choroid is attached to the sclera most firmly round the entrance of the optic nerve. Less firm attachments occur where nerves and vessels enter or leave the choroid. On the inner surface lies the retina, adherent not only at the head of the optic nerve, but also at its anterior edge, the ora serrata. The attachments of the choroid are important when considering its vascularity, for it requires distensibility to enable it to fulfil its function. The presence of the lamina vitrea as its inner boundary probably aids the capacity of the choroid for varying accommodation. The lamina vitrea consists of two layers. An outer layer which is continuous with the elastic fibre network of the choroid, and an inner layer which according to Collins and Mayou (1912) is "a kind of secretion from the pigmented epithelium during embryonic life". The choroid has a certain elasticity. During life it appears to be under tension, for when split there is a definite though not great tendency for it to gape. The rich pigmentation of the whole uveal tract may have for its main function the provision of a dark chamber free from extraneous light and internal reflections. It is interesting to surmise that it also may protect the thin endothelial walls of its concentrated vessels from the ravages of light, and so prevent a consequent increased permeability. The pigment lessens in intensity as the vessels diminish in size from without inwards. The pigmentation does not affect inflammatory changes occurring here, but definitely influences the character of tumour formation.

The vessels are not only very numerous, but their anastomoses are very complex. Vortices are frequent in the layer closest to the retina, the chorio-capillaris. This layer consists almost exclusively of closely packed capillaries with very wide lumina. It is fed directly by the arteries. The region of the choroid opposite the macula is most richly supplied with the smallest capillaries (Parsons). The richness of a plexus of nerves and of ganglion cells has led certain investigators to put the control of the capillaries under its influence. If, as has been assumed, this plexus is composed of sympathetic fibres from the carotid plexus, some explanation can be given for the degree of independence of the intra-ocular capillaries to be referred to later.

THE AQUEOUS: *origin and circulation*. The evidence that the aqueous is a dialysate is convincing. Duke-Elder (1926–7) has demonstrated the similarity of its physical properties, and those of a dialysate of the capillary plasma. If this is so, only two factors can alter its constitution—the composition of the blood, and the permeability of the capillaries. In fact, it is because the aqueous and the capillary plasma are in chemical, hydrostatic, osmotic and electrical equilibrium, and because "there is no evidence of the expenditure of an energy in the elaboration of the one from the other" that Duke-Elder considers the aqueous to be dialysate.

The views put forward to explain the formation of the aqueous have varied from the bestowal on the ciliary body of an active and secretory function (Seidel, 1921; Schmelzer,

1925) to the conception which postulated the uvea as the source of the aqueous and the latter as a fluid stagnant and at rest (Magitot, 1917–22–3–8). For long the filtration theory of Leber (1903), Parsons (1904–8, 1913) and E. E. Henderson and Starling (1906) held the field, but it appears that Duke-Elder's work has established the theory of dialysation through the capillary walls rather than through ciliary epithelium. The injection of dyes into the blood stream, and the study of the consequent *intra vitam* staining of the eye, suggested an almost universal origin from all tissues. The injection of similar dyes into the eye, and a tracing of their paths of exit, suggest wide possibilities of escape. However, as Duke-Elder has shown, these experiments show neither the site of origin, nor of exit, but simply a two-way communication through the capillary walls. "Thus, while a fluid interchange exists throughout the vascularised tissues of the eye as a whole, the location of the greatest pressure-head in the circulation in the distribution of the long posterior ciliary arteries will determine the greatest outward diffusion from the ciliary body and iris; and the position of the canal of Schlemm, far down the venous pressure gradient, with its delicately adjusted pressure equilibrium, will favour a preferential diffusion in the opposite direction at the angle of the anterior chamber" (Duke-Elder).

THE MAINTENANCE OF INTRA-OCULAR PRESSURE. It is essential that a certain intra-ocular pressure should be maintained if the eye is to fulfil its optical function, and if the metabolism of its tissue is to be preserved. The intra-ocular pressure of a normal eye is determined by the hydrostatic pressure in the capillaries minus the difference in osmotic pressure between the aqueous and the capillary plasma.

Intra-ocular pressure may be altered by varying either the blood pressure in the capillaries, or the difference in the osmotic pressure of the aqueous and the capillary plasma, or by a change in the volume of the uveal capillaries, the vitreous or the lens or the quantity of aqueous humour (Duke-Elder).

The blood pressure in the capillaries does not vary

directly with the systemic pressure. This independence is partly due to the control of a local nervous mechanism. It affords a further safeguard for the integrity of the essential vital elements. As capillaries allow a uniform distribution of crystalloids, it is only the relative colloid content of the aqueous and the plasma which can alter the osmotic pressure.

The considerable distensibility of the uveal tract is of great importance. Its variation is a reaction to the "hunger" or to other requirements of the tissues it supplies. The possible variations in the mass of the vitreous and quantity of the aqueous will be considered later. The semi-permeability of the capsule round the lens and the ability of the latter to vary in size are well-known facts. The safety-valve action of the canal of Schlemm is due to the possibility of aqueous escaping through the pectinate ligament when the intra-ocular pressure exceeds that in the exit veins.

THE VITREOUS

The vitreous is a pure homogeneous gel—a colloid solution in which the molecules have set to form a semi-solid jelly. It is unstable, elastic and hydrophylic. In physical properties and in composition it is almost identical with the aqueous—a very dilute sol, that is, a colloid solution in which the molecules are free to move. The essential difference between the two is that the vitreous contains a small amount of mucoprotein for maintaining optical transparency, and a residuary protein, the function of which is gelability. These two constituents, each with a separate function, Duke-Elder considers, are secreted by ectodermal elements mainly in the retina, and are bathed in the common intra-ocular fluid, which dialysing from the capillaries in the ciliary region, percolates through these substances and enters into physical combination with them, thus producing the turgescent gel which forms the vitreous body. The possible variations in turgescence will be considered later.

STRUCTURE AND OPTICAL EFFECTS. Ida Mann, Duke-Elder, Baurmann (1926), Koeppe and others, have demonstrated anatomically and by slit-lamp microscopy, that no containing membrane such as the hyaloid membrane exists. Kraupa (1923–4), Pillat (1922), Isakowitz (1926) and others have described its occurrence in morbid states. Vogt describes it as a pseudo-membrane inserted into the area between the ora serrata and the ciliary processes. In his atlas, he shows it folded as the result of traction when injury had caused vitreous haemorrhage. Mann's and Duke-Elder's researches are convincing, and establish the presence simply of a surface condensation. This appears almost invariably on a colloid, and is associated with the phenomenon of absorption, that is the local condensation of dissolved substances on the surface and between the solid particles and the liquid of the colloid. It depends on the surface tension of the particular colloid.

From their anatomical investigations Salzmann (1912) and E. Fuchs (1912) are satisfied that the vitreous has a framework. In general it has a definite membranous lamellar form, which, as a rule, does not extend anteriorly to the lens surface.

As a result of slit-lamp observations Gullstrand, Vogt (1921), Koeppe (1918), Koby (1920, 1925), Hughes (1929) and others are satisfied that the vitreous is permeated with delicate membranes. Meesmann (1927) in his atlas shows vertical and horizontal band-like effects and delicate dots. Koby, has pointed out that if a large coloboma of the iris is present the vitreous nearest the ciliary region shows a denser framework than elsewhere. This may be due to the different angle of the incident and reflected beams of light. Since using the micro-arc slit-lamp, Vogt is convinced that no vitreous is free of framework, not even in the axial area. But Duke-Elder (1929 a) after investigations with the ultra-microscope wrote that "the apparent texture is an optical delusion, the basis of which is determined by the colloid aggregates although they themselves are too small to be rendered actually visible". They may, he considers, become "optically evident when large numbers of them become arranged in a direction perpendicular to the incident light". It is difficult to distinguish true structure from optical effect. The findings of the histologists "in their preparations bear only a distant resemblance to the living tissues of the vitreous", as Koby has stated; and there is just as great a dissimilarity between the slit-lamp and the ultra-microscopic appearances. Most colloids, unlike molecular solutions, are more or less turbid. They exhibit the Tyndall phenomenon, that is, the colloid particles reflect light from a narrow beam at right angles to them (plane-polarisation) because they are smaller than the mean wave length of the light.

When fresh vitreous is examined by the ultra-microscope it appears optically empty. After several hours minute fibrils appear, such as are seen in soap gels and other colloids. "Under certain conditions, such as alterations in the reaction of the surrounding medium", these fibrillae may break up into a granular form, or may coalesce, giving the appearance of fibres visible by slit-lamp illumination. Occasionally under different conditions the fibrillae may dissolve and disappear. Of the conditions which influence the appearance of these colloid particles, the reaction and the osmotic pressure of the pervading fluid are of the greatest importance. The former depends on the concentration of the dissociated ions, and the latter mainly on concentration of the crystalloids.

TURGESCENCE AND REACTION. When one remembers that the vitreous body occupies four-fifths of the globe, its importance in a consideration of detachment of the retina can be appreciated. Its turgescence must have a definite effect in keeping the retina against the choroid. Its power of absorbing water and swelling up depends mainly on the reaction of the intra-ocular fluid, that is, on the concentration of H ions. The protein of the vitreous is amphoteric and so shares with other proteins the ability to act as an acid or a base, according to whether the NH_2 group or the COOH group is effective; that is whether a negative or a positive electric charge is carried by the protein ion. The turgidity and osmotic pressure are at a minimum when these are balanced, that is at the iso-electric point.

Abé (1927) and Rossier (1928) consider that the vitreous has two or more iso-electric points. Previous workers taking this point to be pH 4·4, found that the normal pH of the vitreous was 7·5–7·7. Therefore the vitreous is more alkaline than the blood. If the pH of the blood or of the vitreous falls and approaches the iso-electric point, the turgescence will lessen and the tension of the eye will fall. It is during such a deturgescence that the fine swollen fibrillae of ultra-microscopic size separate out from solution and coalesce to form fibres of microscopic size, leading to the formation of a curd or coagel. If on the other hand the reaction becomes alkaline, the turgidity, osmotic pressure, and intra-ocular pressure will rise. Duke-Elder's experiments (1929 b) on perfused eyes, have shown that the intra-ocular pressure varies directly with the alterations in the pH of the blood. Here of course the control of systemic influences was eliminated. The variations clinically possible, and the effect of an alteration in the iso-electric point itself, are subjects about which little is proved as yet.

If the turgescence increases, and the semi-solid vitreous requires more space, it acquires this by increasing the pressure in the anterior chamber until it exceeds that in the exit channels, and a loss of aqueous occurs. Blood would also be squeezed out of the choroid. But if the vitreous shrinks, the space is filled partly by aqueous and partly by a choroidal swelling. In this case the retina will not have the same support as it did when solid vitreous pressed it out. It must be remembered that certain observers will not allow that the vitreous plays any but a negligible part in keeping the retina in position. Baurmann states that the pressure of the swelling of the vitreous is only ½–1 mm. of water. He considers that neither this nor any cellular connection between the retina and the pigment epithelium exert a force comparable with that due to the difference in the pressure of the pre-retinal and inter-retinal spaces.

The control of the reaction of the blood is most efficient, depending on the presence of the buffer salts and the response of the respiratory and circulatory systems. Therefore the alterations in pH adopted in experimental work are unlikely to occur in the body, unless under such a local condition as "outlying acidosis". The investigations by Peyton

Rous and Drury (1929) on the question are of great interest. They have shown that an acidosis of the tissues may occur apart from an alteration in the reaction of the blood. When the circulation of a part is seriously impaired, acid substances formed in the tissues tend to be retained. If the blood supply to certain tissues is temporarily cut off or seriously diminished, as for example in serious haemorrhage, this patchy or local acidosis may appear even though unaccompanied by any change in the blood reaction or general blood pressure. When one remembers the supreme control of the capillaries, one realises the possibility of a change in vitreous reaction, due to disordered capillary permeability. That the colloid content of the vitreous can increase if the capillary walls become more permeable has been shown by Guggenheim and Franceschetti (1928).

TURGESCENCE AND OSMOTIC PRESSURE. The fluid content and the turgescence of the vitreous can be influenced by the osmotic pressure of the blood. This, at a given temperature, depends on the concentration of dissolved substances, especially of crystalloids. During life an attempt is made to maintain the osmotic balance constant. Fluid is withdrawn from the tissues in hypertonicity, to lessen the concentration. In hypotonicity the fluid flows in the reverse direction to increase the concentration.

This attempt may explain a fall in tension, and withdrawal of the support to the retina. This is the basis for the osmotic treatment of glaucoma. Hypertonic solutions varying from 10 per cent. to a saturated solution have been given intravenously. Fluid is drawn from all the tissues including those of the eye, and the intra-ocular pressure falls.

Duke-Elder (1929 c) has shown that the volume of the vitreous varies indirectly with the salt content of the blood, and that the presence of sodium chloride has a steadying effect on the influence of an altered reaction. Neither the swelling, which is great with a pH of from 7·5 to 10 on the alkaline side, or of 3 on the acid side, nor the deturgescence of the iso-electric state is as great if the vitreous is in a 15 per cent. saline solution as it would be in one that was salt free.

It is supposed that muscular exertion increases the flow of lymph by breaking down the large molecules in the cell protoplasm into smaller ones. This increases the osmotic pressure and a distension of the cells occurs, due to the absorption of water. By filtration a flow of fluid occurs into the neighbouring lymph spaces (McLeod). Is it possible that some other physical activity can produce an oedema which could cause glaucoma, and that the reverse condition, a dehydration, could by making the vitreous shrink predispose to detachment? Much has yet to be learnt of the possible variations in the crystalloid concentration and the concentration of ions in the fluid bathing the vitreous and lens. Until this has been investigated further, many of the problems of detachment of the retina will remain unsolved.

REACTIONS TO INJURY AND DISEASE. "Normally there is no living cell in the vitreous, and the pathology of this body is largely determined by the cells and cellular products which enter it from adjacent organs" (Friedenwald). Bacteria spreading in from neighbouring parts are free from the inhibiting influence of the tissues. They multiply rapidly, and abscess formation occurs.

Parsons (1929) attributes the ease with which vitreous haemorrhages completely absorb to the absence of meso-blastic tissue. Toxic influences and trauma can cause the liberation of fibroblasts from the mesoblastic tissues surrounding the blood vessels. Once these cells are free, fibrous tissue is formed and the way prepared for the development of retinitis proliferans. Vitreous haemorrhages always absorb more slowly than those in the anterior chamber.

The vitreous is so unstable that it can be broken down by slight mechanical injury. Even filtration and the effect of gravity are sufficient to do this. It slowly passes through ordinary filter paper. Leber was astonished at the appearance of the vitreous after filtration. It can be broken down in a similar manner if suspended from a clamp. The mass slowly breaks down into a clear fluid, leaving suspended the protein of the vitreous as a thin membranous homogeneous film. These reactions are further evidence of the absence of structure in this body. The clinical importance of this is evident when we regard the liquefaction of the vitreous in diseased states, and the appearance in it of fibrillar structures or opacities. Leber's observations on the vitreous compressed by advanced choroidal sarcoma were similar. He found it represented merely by a fibrous layer, about one-fifth of the retinal width.

REFERENCES

THE RETINA AND THE CHOROID

1877. DONDERS, F. C. *Arch. f. Ophthal.* **23**, 255.
1888. KERSCHBAUMER. *Ibid.* **34**, 16.
1892. —— *Ibid.* **38**, 127.
1893. CAJAL, RAMÓN Y. "La Rétine des Vertébrés", *La Cellule*, **9**.
1900. GREEF, R. *Graefe-Saemisch Handb. d. ges. Augenheilk.* 2nd edn., part 1, **1**, chap. 5.
1907. SALZMANN, M. "On the Anatomy and Pathology of Keratoconus", *Arch. f. Ophthal.* **67**, 1.
1910. HALBEN, R. *Die Kopulation der Netzhaut mit der Aderhaut durch Kontaktverbindung*, Berlin.
1912. COLLINS, E. TREACHER and MAYOU, M. S. *Pathology. Pyle's System*, 1st edn., 481.
1912. SALZMANN, M. *The Anatomy and Histology of the Human Eye*, Leipzig.
1918. KOEPPE, L. *Arch. f. Ophthal.* **97**, 346.
1919. FUSITA. *Nippon Gank. Zasshi.* Aug.
1919. OGUCHI, C. *Ibid.* July.
1920. EBBECKE, E. *Deut. phys. Gesell.* Hamburg meeting.
1920. FERREE, C. E. and RAND, G. *Amer. Jl. of Phys. Optics*, **1**, 185; *Amer. Jl. of Ophthal.* (abstract), **3**, 272.
1920. SAKAI. *Nippon Gank. Zasshi.* July.
1922. KROGH, A. *The Anatomy and Physiology of the Capillaries*, New Haven.
1923. SPALTEHOLZ, W. *Klin. Monatsbl. f. Augenheilk.* **71**, 246.
1924. BRYSON, L. H. *Reports of St Andrew's Institute for Clinical Research*, **3**, 35.
1924. EGGER, A. *Arch. f. Ophthal.* **113**, 1.
1924. FRIEDENWALD, J. S. *Amer. Jl. of Ophthal.* **7**, 940.
1924. v. HELMHOLTZ, H. *Treatise of Phys. Optics*, **2**, 10, trans. by Southall.
1924. LUNDSGAARD, K. K. *Acta Ophthal.* **2**, 112.
1924. POSKROWSKY. *Klin. Monatsbl. f. Augenheilk.* **72**, 289.
1925. FRIEDENWALD, J. S. *Amer. Jl. of Ophthal.* **8**, 177.
1925. OGUCHI, C. *Arch. f. Ophthal.* **115**, 234.

1926. AREY, L. B. *Jl. of Compar. Anat.* **26**, 213.
1926 OGUCHI, C. *Arch. f. Ophthal.* **117**, 208.
1926. SCHEERER, R. *Klin. Monatsbl. f. Augenheilk.* **76**, 524.
1926. SUGITA, Y. *Arch. f. Ophthal.* **116**, 653.
1928. MANN, IDA. *The Development of the Human Eye*, Cambridge.
1929. MAITLAND RAMSAY, A. *The Eye in General Medicine*, London, p. 10.
1929. TRANTAS, A. *Arch. d'Ophtal.* **46**, 551.
1929. WOOD-JONES, F. and PORTEUS, S. D. *The Matrix of the Mind*, London, 1929.
1930. FORTIN, E. *Klin. Monatsbl. f. Augenheilk.* **84**, 136.
1930. FUCHS, E. *Arch. of Ophthal.* **3**, 396.

THE AQUEOUS

1903. LEBER, TH. *Graefe-Saemisch Handb. d. ges. Augenheilk.* 2nd edn., **2**, 207.
1904–8. PARSONS, J. H. *The Pathology of the Eye*, London, **3**.
1906. HENDERSON, E. E. and STARLING, E. H. *Proc. Roy. Soc.* Ser. B, **77**, 294.
1913. PARSONS, J. H. *Proc. Roy. Soc. Med.* **6**, 3.
1917. MAGITOT, A. *Ann. d'Ocul.* **154**, 65.
1921. SEIDEL, E. *Arch. f. Ophthal.* **104**, 284.
1922. MAGITOT, A. *Ann. d'Ocul.* **159**, 401.
1923. —— *Ibid.* **160**, 18.
1925. SCHMELZER. *Ber. ü. d. Versamml. d. deutsch. ophthal. Gesellsch.* 259.
1926. DUKE-ELDER, W. S. *Brit. Jl. of Ophthal.* **10**, 513.
1927. —— "The Nature of the intra-ocular Fluids", *Brit. Jl. of Ophthal.* Monograph Supplement, **3**.
1926–7. —— *Jl. of Physiol.* **62**, 315.
1928. —— *Ibid.* **64**, 78.
1928. MAGITOT, A. *Ann. d'Ocul.* **165**, 481.

THE VITREOUS

1912. FUCHS, E. *Arch. f. Ophthal.* **99**, 202.
1912. SALZMANN, M. *Anatomy and Histology of the Human Eye*, 150.
1918. KOEPPE, L. *Arch. f. Ophthal.* **97**, 198.
1920. KOBY, F. E. *Rev. gén. d'Ophtal.* April, **34**, 160.
1921. VOGT, A. *Atlas of Microscopy of the Living Eye*, trans. by von der Heydt, Berlin.
1922. PILLAT, A. *Klin. Monatsbl. f. Augenheilk.* **69**, 429.
1923. KRAUPA, E. *Ibid.* **70**, 716.
1924. —— *Ibid.* **72**, 476.
1925. KOBY, F. E. *Slit-lamp Microscopy of the Living Eye*, trans. by Goulden and Harris, London.
1926. BAURMANN, M. *Arch. f. Ophthal.* **117**, 304.

1926. Isakowitz, J. *Klin. Monatsbl. f. Augenheilk.* **77**, 121.

1927. Abé, T. *Arch. de Physique Biol.* 6th Jan.

1927. Meesmann, A. *Atlas of Microscopy of the Living Eye*, Berlin, Plates 186–190.

1928. Guggenheim, I. and Franceschetti, A. *Arch. f. Augenheilk.* **98**, 448.

1928. Rossier, H. *Ann. de Méd.* **23**, 348.

1929 a. Duke-Elder, W. S. *Trans. Ophthal. Soc. U.K.* **49**, 84, 88, 100.

1929 b. —— *Brit. Jl. of Ophthal.* **13**, 385.

1929 c. —— *Trans. Ophthal. Soc. U.K.* **49**, 100

1929. Hughes, N. *Ibid.* **49**, 407.

1929. Parsons, Sir John. *Ibid.* **49**, 193.

1929. Peyton Rous and Drury. *Jl. of Expt. Med.* 1st March.

CHAPTER III

PATHOGENESIS

In attempting to understand the origin and development of retinal detachment, we must consider the ocular changes with which we find it associated. At the same time we must attempt to exclude those that are purely secondary and degenerative, and therefore unlikely to throw light on the mechanism which has caused the detachment. Gonin (1919) wisely attributes the large percentage of failures in treatment to the fact that the mechanism producing the separation is so poorly understood. In each case an endeavour must be made to ascertain the exact mechanism at work. For this purpose the early clinical findings, the histological examination of recent detachments, and experimental research can help us most. It has been customary for continental writers to consider the causes of detachment of the retina under four headings. Formerly each heading was synonymous with a separate theory. Though less importance is attached now to certain of these theories, it is convenient to consider the pathogenesis in this way. By so doing, most of the main aetiological factors can be introduced. The essential value of certain of these is simply in the fact that they were stepping-stones to research, which has helped to elucidate the problem. The four theories are those of Distension, Depression, Attraction, Exudation.

THE THEORY OF DISTENSION

(*a*) ASSOCIATION OF MYOPIA. Early observers were interested in the preponderance of myopes amongst patients with detachment of the retina. They considered the stretching of the choroid and sclera to be the actual cause of the retinal separation. Later it will be shown that this is only an indirect relationship. Graefe (1857) estimated that from 50 to 66 per cent. of spontaneous detachments occurred in myopes. He believed that if the retina was not sufficiently extensible, the increase in length of the axis of vision in myopia could produce a separation of retina from choroid. Parsons (1904–8 a), in his *Pathology of the Eye* states that detachment of the retina occurs in all grades of myopia, especially above 13 dioptres. Leber compiled statistics which summarised twelve series published by various oculists between 1879 and 1914, and he found that of 3408 eyes with detachment of the retina, 2219 or 65·1 per cent. were myopic. Helming (1915), in his series of 162 unilateral and 9 bilateral detachments of the retina, found myopia as the only apparent cause in 33 per cent. In 6 cases lens extraction for myopia had been done; in 4 of them many years before. Seible (1916), in a series of 163 detachments of the retina, found 92 were myopic, and of these 61 were over 7 D. In 64 myopia appeared to be the only cause; in 20 trauma was an additional factor, and in 15 iridocyclitis was present. In Schreiber's series (1920), of 186 eyes in the Heidelberg Clinic, 69 were considered to be due to myopia. A great number of myopic cases showing exudative processes in the uvea were excluded. In Uhthoff's series (1922) myopia was given as the cause in 61 per cent. Galezowski collected 1158 cases of detachment of the retina, and of these 918 were in myopes, or almost 80 per cent. If two-thirds of retinal detachments occur in myopes, let us consider the proportion of myopes which develop this condition. Horstmann, in a series of 3581 myopic eyes, found 125 with detachment, or 3·5 per cent. Schleich found it in 2·6 per cent. of 1156 eyes. Hertel in 0·96 per cent., and Proskauer in 0·71 per cent. That it is more common in the higher degrees of myopia is the conclusion of von Hippel (1899), and Otto (1897), who found it respectively in 6·7 and 5·9 per cent. of eyes with over 10 D. of myopia. Nordenson showed that in a series of 97 detachments, in 26·3 per cent. the myopia was below 6 D., and in 30·7 per cent. above 6 D. Now as myopia occurs in 15 per cent. of otherwise healthy eyes, in a low degree, it is almost twice as frequent in eyes with detachment of the retina. Therefore the factor which makes these eyes susceptible to detachment must exist even in the lower degrees of myopia. According to Horstmann's statistics, amongst myopes with from 2–4 D., 19 detachments were found; from 4–6 D., 10 cases; from 6–8 D., 10 cases; 8–10 D., 17 cases; and over 10 D., 26 cases. This means 39 amongst myopes with less than 8 D., and 43 amongst those with more than 8 D. To realise the tremendous disproportion, one must remember the relative infrequency of myopia of over 8 D.

PATHOLOGY OF MYOPIA. "It has been estimated that the area of the fundus posterior to the equator in the normal eye measures about 9 sq. cm.; this is increased from 4 to 6 sq. cm. in an eye 31 mm. in length" (Parsons, 1904–8 b). Hanssen's work (1925) on this subject is very interesting. He has proved that the stretching of the myopic eye is not simply near the posterior pole. In a series of specimens, the breadth of the ciliary region, as measured from the anterior insertion of the ciliary muscle to the ora serrata, was from 6·6 to 10 mm. In a similar series of normal eyes, the measurements were from 5 to 6 mm. and never more than 7. In a series of 37 eyes examined microscopically, marked thinning of the retina was found in 26, and in 16 of these it was in the anterior segment close to the ora serrata. Actual hole formation was found in many of these eyes. The distensibility of the choroid lying within the very inelastic sclera and the relative inelasticity of the retina are striking facts. There is a potential space between the choroid and sclera, and between the inner and outer retinal layers. The choroid is separated from the outer retinal layer by a thin elastic membrane, the lamina vitrea, or the membrane of Bruch.

In myopia the capacity of the eye increases, but if Duke-Elder is correct, there is no increase in the amount of normal vitreous or renewal if any is lost. So fluid fills up the remaining space. As the sclera and choroid stretch, the normal fine relations between the retinal pigment epithelium and the rods and cones are broken down. The vitreous becomes degenerate and the retina atrophic. This eye is now susceptible to toxic influences or circulatory disturbances which make for effusion or haemorrhage, and to trauma or exertion which can easily cause rents or apertures in the degenerate retina. A consideration of the causes of myopia may throw light on the most probable mechanism which will relate these lesions to a separation of the retina.

CAUSES OF MYOPIA. Von Graefe was inclined to consider that the distension of the sclera and choroid, characteristic of myopia, was the cause of this striking association of myopia and detachment of the retina. We must remember that his conception of the cause of myopia receives little support now. According to Fuchs, his view was that an inflammation of the posterior scleral and choroidal tissues, "scleroticochoroiditis posterior", led to a stretching similar to an ectasia in the ciliary region. More recently Maitland Ramsay has expressed similar views which can be summarised as follows:

All changes in myopia are due to inflammation of the choroid at the posterior pole. These changes lead to a weakening of the overlying sclera, which, yielding to intra-ocular pressure, bulges backwards to form a posterior staphyloma. The mechanism of production is similar to that of a ciliary ectasia, due to prolonged anterior sclerotico-choroiditis. The retina displaced by inflammatory exudate deprived of its natural support, owing to the fluidity and shrinking of the vitreous, becomes detached. There is widespread opposition to this view. The general opinion is against the idea that myopia can be explained on an inflammatory basis. Therefore it would be wise to consider more probable explanations.

Parsons has stated that "the condition of the choroid in the grosser changes of myopia is one of stretching and atrophy, with little or no evidence of inflammation". Salzmann found defects in the lamina elastica in the affected areas; they appeared as clefts and they were attributed to stretching. Such tears may lead to proliferation of the pigment epithelium and cicatrisation differing in no way from the scarring following choroiditis; hence the great similarity in the ophthalmoscopic appearances. The scars themselves lead to fresh tears owing to their resistance and lack of elasticity, so that the changes are progressive. The chief change in the choroid itself is the disappearance of the lumina of the vessels. The retinal changes are wholly secondary to those in the choroid. They are at first limited to the outer layers which are dependent upon the chorio-capillaris for nutrition. Failure of blood supply in this layer leads to the same changes as those seen in retinitis pigmentosa and choroiditis. The retinal atrophy usually ceases with the outer reticular layer, as the inner layers of the retina are supplied by the retinal vascular system. Fusion with the choroid occurs where the lamina elastica is defective, as in disseminated choroiditis (Parsons).

Fuchs states that straining at near work in youth is probably the main cause of myopia. There are other additional factors, viz. (a) anatomical predisposition, e.g. defective resistance of sclera and peculiarities in relations of muscles, optic nerve and choroid. These are always apt to be hereditary, and so this tendency is readily accounted for; (b) circumstances which compel too great approximation to work, e.g. insufficient illumination, particularly fine work, and a diminution of visual acuity by astigmatism and corneal and lenticular opacities. The stretching is in reality an exaggerated normal process. It is due to a disproportion between the natural elongating force and the resistance offered to it by the coats of the eye. The part played by defective resistance is probably the greater. The following are the main theories propounded to explain the elongation:

1. A congenital defect which causes reduced rigidity of coats of eye (Schnabel). Salzmann held that the stretching of the choroid was passive, following the bulging of an insufficiently resisting sclera, and that the tears in the lamina vitrea were spontaneous and not secondary to atrophy of the chorio-capillaris (Parsons).

2. An increase in intra-ocular tension due to physiological effort (Edridge Green).

3. The pressure on the eyeball by muscles, especially by the obliques during convergence, causes a rise in intra-ocular pressure. This is aided by venous congestion due to the muscles pressing on the venae vorticosae (Stilling). Ochi adds to this a congenitally weak sclera.

4. The poor development of the ciliary muscle. A. Wood considers this to be the cause, and not the result of myopia.

Thomson believed that the ciliary muscle aids the outflow of the aqueous, and, if it is not sufficiently strong, there is a retarded flow, a rise in intra-ocular pressure which causes distension of the coats of the eye in early life.

5. The rapid growth of the retina. Vogt considers that if the retina extends too rapidly, its protective coverings stretch and atrophy.

6. Certain authors, remembering the effect on the choroid which the meridional fibres of the ciliary muscles have, as the tensor choroidae, state that if the nutrition of the elastic tissue of the eye is affected, especially that of the lamina vitrea—stretching, atrophy and splitting will ensue (Newman, 1929).

Comberg (1928) has shown that there is a vibration of the posterior pole when reading, and a backward pushing of the eye when the lids are opened and closed. The push of the lids when blinking, corresponds to varying weights, 15–20 grm. These two factors make for distension in the posterior pole. Thorner, years before, stated that the harmful effect of reading was due to the associated quick jerking movements.

Levinsohn (1928) considers that the position of the head and the effect of gravity is of greater danger. This, he states, will explain the much greater frequency of myopia amongst type-setters than amongst watch-makers. After experiments in which he developed myopia in monkeys' eyes by keeping their heads downwards, he concluded that heredity is only a determining factor, and that the abuse of eyes in ordinary daily life is the main factor.

At birth the sclera is immature, and is particularly lacking in elastic fibres, and until the beginning of the third decade, it is particularly poor in elastic tissue. From then on, until the age of sixty years, this increases greatly (Krekler, 1923). Thinness alone of the sclera is not sufficient for the development of myopia, for, if it were, most patients with "blue sclerotics" would be myopic. Anatomical support is wanting for the following theories—low orbital index with vertical pressure on the growing eye, long orbit or relatively short optic nerve, abnormal interpupillary distance and excessive divergence of the orbits. As time goes by, it appears as if an inherited weakness of the sclera, possibly accentuated by overuse or abuse of eyes for near work, is the most probable explanation of myopia.

The great significance of inheritance is emphasised by most of these theories though in different ways. "The changes in the retina and in the choroid that occur in the neighbourhood of the papilla in cases of myopia are caused not so much by mechanical effects, as people used to believe, but rather they represent an ontogenetic process predetermined by phylogenetic processes and influences" (Clausen 1928).

OBJECTIONS TO THIS THEORY. Leber objected to this theory because he considered that the retina was as extensible as the choroid and the sclera. His observations of choroidal tears after contusions when the retina remained intact, and of the absence of detachment in many advanced myopic staphylomata appeared to support this. He considered that the retina would tear rather than detach when the limit of extensibility was passed, because the fluid producing the dilatation was pressing from within and tending to keep the retina in place.

More importance should be attached to the fact that numbers of patients with detachment of the retina are not myopic. It is important to realise too that when the actual separation occurs spontaneously the patient is usually over fifty years of age, whilst the progressive and dangerous period in myopia is under thirty. This suggests that the cause of myopia, whatever its nature, is not, as a rule, simultaneously causing detachment of the retina. If there is a tendency for the retina to leave a stretched choroid, it cannot be great, otherwise it would do so frequently in staphyloma and buphthalmia. The detachment of the retina must be due to some delayed effect, or secondary degeneration.

If the separation is due to the distension *per se*, why is the proportion of detachments of the retina in eyes with extreme myopia not much greater? Probably retino-choroidal adhesions prevent the separation of the two layers. The adherence of the choroid to the pigment epithelium in myopia is of interest. Dor (1921) considered that there is even a protective antagonism between detachment of the retina and posterior sclero-choroiditis. He rarely found detachment of the retina in myopic posterior-choroiditis, and when it did occur, it was usually curable by subconjunctival injections. Lauber (1923) considered that the adhesions forming in such eyes might limit the spread of the detachment of the retina. Meller agrees with this view. He has frequently found with the microscope small detachments of the retina in similar eyes. They appeared to be limited by adhesions. Sometimes, owing to the presence of such adhesions, or to the formation of cystic spaces, the outer layers of the retina may remain attached to the choroid and only the inner layers be found detached. Gilbert (1920), as a result of his histological study of myopic eyes, stated that, when the lamina vitrea and pigment epithelium degenerate, adhesions between the retina and choroid are formed. At some of these sites the retina appeared to be drawn into the defects in the choroid. Fuchs's finding (1920) that the retina was completely detached in a myopic eye, except where it was adherent to the choroid in a staphylomatous cup, is of interest. This and the fact that the chorio-capillaris is atrophic suggests that vascular exudation, which will be considered later, is of little importance in detachments in myopia.

Though choroidal changes are commonly in direct relation to the degree of myopia, the risk of detachment does not appear to vary directly. In a series of 304 patients, Rehsteiner (1928) found peripheral lesions in 26 per cent. of those with from 1 to 10 D. of myopia, 50 per cent. of those with 11 to 20 D., and 75 per cent. of those with over 20 D. In anisometropia only the myopic eye showed the areas of degeneration. Salzmann states that the choroidal degeneration in myopia is directly proportional to the degree of myopia, but that there is no relationship between the latter factor and the presence or absence of detachment of the retina. He considers that myopia may itself be due to relaxation of the suspensory ligament when the orbiculus ciliaris becomes detached.

We can conclude therefore that the association is not simply due to the elongation of the eye, on the assumption that the inelastic retina takes the chord of the arc (the stretched sclera and choroid) which it cannot describe, but that the relationship probably depends on some associated degeneration in the retina, choroid, vitreous and ciliary body. If the stretching of the retina is not the direct cause of the separation from the choroid, it may play an indirect rôle by leading to degeneration and hole formation.

CYSTOID DEGENERATION OF THE RETINA (v. Plate 2 a). Hanssen (1925) considers that the spontaneous detachments in myopic and senile eyes are due to alterations in the retina. The following findings amongst others force him to consider a retinal tear to be the necessary preliminary condition. Of thirty-seven myopic eyes, free from detachments, twenty-six showed partial retinal atrophy, cystoid degeneration, tears in the inner layers and actual holes. In sixteen eyes this occurred in the anterior area, and of these four showed fissures, and six showed holes. In six, changes were found in the equatorial region. His work (1925) on myopic degeneration proves the existence of cystoid retinal degeneration as a common condition. It occurs not only in normal senile eyes, but also in early life in the periphery of myopic eyes. A degeneration of retinal elements occurs with the collection of highly albuminous fluid. This is followed by the formation of cysts. If these become atrophic, holes in the retina may form, and these may play an important part in the production of a detachment. Fuchs (1921) agrees with this view. It is however in opposition to the older view that the cysts were primary and not due to degeneration. Apart from cysts associated with glaucoma, Fuchs considers those on the outer retinal surface to be due to inflammation of retina and choroid, and those on the inner surface to traction by vitreous bands, or shrinking retinal membranes. If a cyst is covered simply by the internal limiting membrane, a slight injury can produce a tear. Hanssen considers that this mechanism accounts for the majority of spontaneous detachments of the retina. Additional factors, he thinks, are the vitreous changes, emphasised as essential by Koeppe, Comberg, Vogt and others, and the reduced tension of the myopic eye.

Gonin (1921) was one of the first to dispel the belief that the cysts were merely degenerative and secondary to a detachment. He found them in recent detachments, and emphasised their rôle as the cause of the condition. Vogt, Kalt and others have seen cysts and punched-out holes or tears in the same fundus as a detached retina. These cysts were found regularly in normal eyes of old people, and at an earlier age and to a more marked degree in axial myopia. As a rule the holes are too peripheral to be clearly seen with the ophthalmoscope. The associated pigment areas and white atrophic changes are visible. Gonin (1919) states that degenerative retinal changes, especially hole formation, are in themselves sufficient to cause detachment of the retina. It is not necessary to assume proliferation of a membrane. He considers that even large areas of peripheral choroidal atrophy with hole formation and detachment of the retina may occur as a result of the vascular degeneration of senility, apart from any infection. Ochi states that these cysts may be seen after death when the retina becomes opaque. They appear as dark areas on the greyish retina in the neighbourhood of the ora serrata. It is necessary to consider the supposed cause of these lesions.

An oedema or a cystoid degeneration. Various opinions have been held regarding cystoid degeneration in the periphery of the retina. While Müller (1857) was the first to describe it, he considered it a post-mortem change. Henle was the first to demonstrate its frequent occurrence. Blessig (1855) considered it to be normal and called the spaces cysts. Iwanoff (1865) held that it was a morbid change and due to oedema. He did not find it in twenty globes of children under eight years of age, but in 12 per cent. of eyes from patients between twenty and forty years, and in 50 per cent. of eyes between fifty and eighty years. Nettleship (1876) described it as "cystic disease" and not as an oedema. Greeff (1900) and Salzmann (1912) considered that it could occur in youth, and was then due to some circulatory

PLATE II

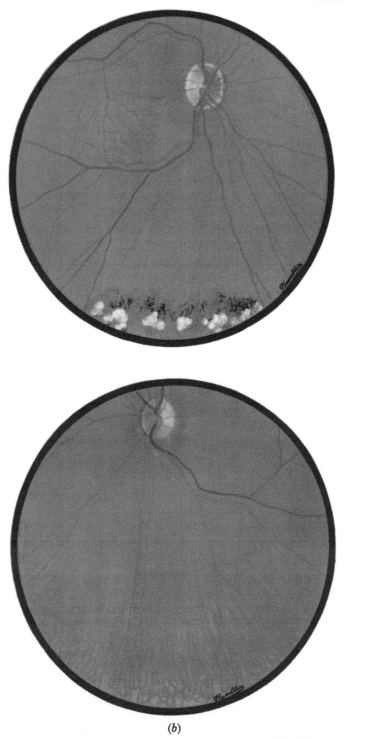

(b)

(a) Peripheral cystoid degeneration (partly diagrammatic). (b) Normal
fundus, drawn as far as the ora serrata (partly diagrammatic).

disturbance. In common with most German writers, they refer to the condition as "cystoid" degeneration. It was soon found that degenerations of this kind are not exclusively limited to the ora serrata. Berger (1924), describing it as "Iwanoff's retinal oedema", states that it is primarily an oedema due to capillary degeneration. Ochi (1927) found this degeneration not only in myopes and in the eyes of the elderly, as Hanssen had, but also in children. In a series of fifteen children under five years of age, where death was due to various causes, it occurred three times. Pressburger (1929) found that the cystoid changes could occur at any age and that they began in the inner granular layer; that they were so peripheral that only once did they appear more than 7 mm. from the ora serrata. He considered that the pull of the vitreous on this area of the retina contributed to cyst and hole formation. If then this condition, which may predispose to retinal separation, can occur at any age, it may account for such an accident not only in the myopic but also in the senile eye.

The periphery of the retina is most affected by this degeneration, for several reasons. Histologically it is an area of transition. Any interference with the retinal circulation will be first felt here, because it is the distal extremity of the retina. Ochi considers that this area is liable to degenerative changes, because it is close to the ora serrata which is adherent to the vitreous, and because it may be influenced by strain of the ciliary muscles and the zonule of Zinn. Salzmann considers that the first traces of cystoid degeneration appear early in life and immediately behind the ora serrata. There is a degeneration of cells with the formation of irregular spaces which later form smooth-walled cavities. The larger cysts may reach so close to the external limiting membrane that at most a layer of outer nuclei remains. On the inner surface remnants of the nerve fibre layer and the internal limiting membrane persist. The walls of partition between the neighbouring cysts become narrower and the thickness of the retina may be doubled. The changes are so common as to be considered physiological. They are not necessarily senile, for they may be very advanced by the end of the fourth decade. A surface view reveals these cysts as isolated or confluent rounded pores separated by narrow partitions. Kapuczinski's recent paper (1929) appears to confirm Vogt's contention that cystoid degeneration is the primary cause of detachment in senility and myopia. Areas of cystoid degeneration lie usually too close to the ora serrata to be seen with the ophthalmoscope. More frequently one can see the pigmented areas and bright white areas of retino-choroidal atrophy which are associated changes.

This discussion has led us far from the question of distension. It appears however that, in so far as distension leads to atrophic retinal areas and degeneration of the vitreous and the uvea, it may play a part in the production of detachment of the retina.

(b) ASSOCIATION OF TRAUMA. The majority agree that violent distension due to trauma is likely to cause a detachment of the retina. Many cases of avulsion or dialysis of the retina from the orbiculus ciliaris at the ora serrata have been reported. They are usually due to trauma and they are often not found by ophthalmoscopic examination, because of vitreous haemorrhages (Scheffels, 1891; Martin, 1929; Fuchs, 1920). A posterior dialysis or avulsion from the optic nerve is much rarer. Gonin has demonstrated a series of twelve eyes of undoubted retinal rupture at the ora, due to sudden distension.

If perforating injuries are excluded, Leber considered that trauma played a part in from 16 to 18 per cent. of retinal detachments. Just as one must guard against statements that are too absolute concerning the influence of myopia, one must also refrain from attaching too much importance to the effect of injury. A patient can usually find some injury in the past if he is asked whether such ever did occur, no matter what the lesion under investigation.* On the other hand, Leber

* The question of liability and compensation arises here. A complete series could be described in which trauma plays a varying part. At one end of the series there are detachments due to direct ocular injury, and to indirect trauma, either as one concentrated blow or effort, or a series of vibrations, and at the other end those due to vibrations that one can class as physiological movements of the body, viz. spontaneous detachments.

One must consider the authenticity of the patient's statements, and the years ago emphasised the slight traction that was sufficient to detach a retina. In an eye, predisposed to retinal detachment by the presence of a retinal hole or of vitreous degeneration, even slight injury may be sufficient to produce the separation. Apparently unrelated falls, light blows on eye or head may be sufficient. Vogt has described detachments which developed during or soon after gymnastic exercises, massage of the eye, and the multiple vibrations of long train or motor journeys. The ages of the three patients who developed detachment during journeys were forty-five, forty-five and sixty years, and the degree of myopia 7, 5, 6 D. One of these was a medical man with 6 D. of myopia, who developed a detachment in his only useful eye immediately after a train journey. The other eye had been blind from a similar lesion for some time. Two maternal aunts, also elderly myopes, were blind from bilateral spontaneous detachments.

We cannot ignore slight trauma whether direct or indirect. That an indirect trauma can cause a detachment of the retina may be proved by a remarkable diversity of cases. A patient reported by Lacroix (1919) showed an unusual appearance. A man received a blow on the upper lid with a piece of wood. Two weeks later when the vitreous had cleared, two tears were found, and a retinal vein was found to be detached from a normal area of retina, and lying loose in

tendency, on finding a defect, to think "Did I injure it?" If possible, collateral evidence should be obtained. One must remember that a detachment may be delayed and occur years after an injury—a fact stressed by Gifford. One must admit that bodily exertion, and not necessarily actual trauma, may produce a detachment. If this occurs during the regular pursuit of occupation, such as when a man lifts a heavy weight, or slips when carrying a sack of grain, the lesion is due to his work. One must be very guarded if the detachment appears only after some time has elapsed since such an occurrence. Then we must decide whether the trauma in question was a factor *sine qua non*, or an irrelevant incident. In the highly degenerate eye of the myope the appearance of a detachment may be excited by a trivial injury. Indeed the trauma often plays a very small part in the production of such a lesion, but it is the exciting part. In these cases partial compensation is the fairest treatment. We must not forget detachments that occur years after the magnetic extraction of minute foreign bodies, or after the removal of a traumatic cataract. For further consideration of this question see Vogt (1929) and Cords (1930).

the vitreous. A patient reported by Vogt (1919) gave an interesting story. He was a myope who developed a detachment of the retina when a train started suddenly. Reattachment and complete visual return followed rest in bed for a year. The relationship of vibration and the onset of detachment has been fully discussed by Breuckner (1919). Neblett (1924) describes a detachment which occurred in the eye of an air pilot during a tail spin. The strain on the patient during a dental extraction has been considered a cause of detachment (McDavitt, 1920). Detachments have been described following the lifting of heavy weights, abdominal straining, and efforts that produced head hyperaemia (Ammann, 1919). Dubois and Cuperus (1921), Rochat (1919), and Francisco (1918), amongst others, have described blows on the back of the head which have led to detachment of the retina. Francisco's case is worthy of mention. After a fall from a bicycle, a man was unconscious for ten days, and each eye showed extensive retinal detachment. After four months' medical treatment recovery was complete. The development of these detachments can be understood when we remember the damage that can be caused to the macula and the surrounding region, as a result of injuries to the skull. Thirty or more distinct patches of exudate may be seen, or if confluent a continuous layer appears. The white areas are due to collections of lymph between the inner retinal surface and the membrana limitans interna. Purtscher, in 1910, described this condition as "traumatic retinal angiopathy", and others since then have confirmed the appearance (Stähli, 1915). Vogt and Knuesel (1921), when reporting three examples, gave a review of the literature to date (Chou, 1929).

One must remember that a detachment of the retina can occur several months or even years after the injury. Reese (1925) reported a detached retina which followed an injury that had taken place three years before. Brinton (1922), Gifford and La Rue (1922) mention similar examples. Gifford for this reason advises bandaging for at least a week after any severe contusion, and the avoidance of violent exercise for two years. He considers haemorrhages or opaque areas in the periphery as danger signals. It appears therefore that the actual effect of any trauma is difficult to gauge, and its results may be very delayed.

THE MECHANISM OF TRAUMA. It is necessary to consider briefly the varying effects of trauma on the eye. They will vary according to the size and velocity of the body causing trauma, and the site of impact.

If the sclera is struck, but not perforated, by a comparatively slowly moving object, as is common in civil life, three areas appear to be most vulnerable. (a) The superior medial quadrant. Usually the direction of the blow is from the front or downwards and outwards, and if the sclera ruptures, it is in this region, 3 mm. posterior to the limbus. This area is the least supported at the moment of impact. Rauber, in his experiments, found that the resistance of an envelope to pressure is one-third greater than its tensile strength. Therefore the eyeball yields at some distance from the site of pressure application. Though the sclera is supported at the site of impact, and ruptures some distance away, the retina is frequently found torn here. The retina may also tear elsewhere due to the distension in the equator of the globe round the line of impact. (b) The retina opposite the site of impact. The strongest wave of pressure due to the blow—the incident wave—will meet the reflected wave at a point just within the sclera, and opposite the site of impact. As a result, the pressure is greatly increased at this spot, and retinal rupture can occur here by contre-coup. At times the choroid only is torn and the commonest site for this to occur is close to the optic disc, and usually on the temporal side. The tear is curved, with its concavity towards the disc. Leber pointed out that the retina usually remains intact over these tears. If the retina is affected its injury takes the form of a macular hole. Leber could collect only four cases where the retina and the choroid in the neighbourhood of the optic nerve were torn in the same place (Cowell, 1869; Gonin, 1912; Hughes, 1887; Graefe, 1854). It is more usual to find a rupture of the anterior choroid associated with a retinal tear in the same vicinity. It is surprising on first thought that the delicate retina should escape when the elastic choroid tears. It is partly because the retina and the choroid are not closely connected, and because the choroid is firmly fixed to the sclera by numerous vessels and nerves. The ductility of the nerve-fibre layer and the presence of the blood vessels give the retina further support. (c) The third area found affected after such injuries is the macular area. It is the most delicate part of the retina, and that which is least protected by a framework of blood vessels. The innermost layer of ductile nerve fibres is also absent. The ductility of these fibres is shown by their maintenance of integrity in papilloedema. This capacity for stretching must afford the retina some protection. So the absence of the nerve-fibre layer at the macula means a lowered resistance to the influence of trauma. The lesions which appear at the sites mentioned vary. They include commotio retinae, haemorrhages, retinal tears and detachments, and choroidal ruptures.

Remarkable instances occurred during the war of bullets which, traversing the orbit and missing the eyeball, produced considerable damage by concussion. The areas affected were again those close to the site of impact or the path of the missile, those opposite this site, and the macular region. For further information on these changes Sir William Lister's excellent articles (1924) should be consulted.

If the missile, which strikes the eye, is moving with great velocity, and does not destroy the globe completely, the sclera will probably be perforated. If the missile is small it meets with little resistance, and apart from perforation, no rupture will occur. But if the object has sufficient size and velocity to overcome the elasticity of the coats of the globe, widespread ruptures will occur. The actual site of rupture will vary according to the site of perforation.

Sometimes a small foreign body, which has perforated the anterior tissues, reaches the retina and its force is spent. It may adhere at the site where it reaches the retina, or it may fall down and become encapsulated near the lower pole. In such cases a tear may occur, directly or as a result of the contraction of fibrous tissue which forms and drags on the retina. In Lister's classical case, a foreign body struck the retina and rebounded twice, coming to rest far forward in the vitreous. The two scars on the retina due to the two impacts of the foreign body produced two scotomata in the visual field.

RETINAL TEARS. Later it will appear that neither the fibrillary vitreous degeneration nor the preretinitis of Leber will explain the vast majority of senile and myopic detachments. As hole formation is common to both theories considered so far, and as retinal tears are considered to be primary by such brilliant modern observers as Vogt and Gonin, we must consider more fully the appearance and causes of such apertures. As a rule a hole in the retina appears as a red area, darker than the normal fundus, lying in a grey area of detached retina. Tears are often gaping, with everted edges. Early the edge appears oedematous. As the retina degenerates, a tear becomes difficult to see. Elschnig (1914) has watched a hole develop. He has described a detached area of retina which became less grey in one part, and later red, as it became thinner and the choroid showed through the hole which appeared. Since Vogt's description of grey areas as holes and of holes with "lids" (see later) this observation is of great interest. Elschnig considered that autolytic ferments in the subretinal fluid produced this destruction. Holes also may be caused by the breakdown of adhesions due to previous inflammation.

FREQUENCY OF TEARS. De Wecker (1870) appears to have been the first to emphasise the frequent occurrence of tears in spontaneous detachment of the retina. Leber (1916) stated that in every case of spontaneous and sudden detachment of the retina, a tear was to be expected. In a series of twenty-seven, he found tears in fourteen. They were considerably more common in recent detachments (73 per cent.) than in those of over two months' duration (about 45 per cent.). Probably there is a tendency for the edges to heal, and the atrophy of the retina makes them invisible as time passes. Leber, Schweigger, Horstmann and Sattler described instances in which this had occurred. Once the subretinal fluid sinks to the lower half of the fundus, and the upper part of the retina begins to re-attach, the tear becomes increasingly difficult to see. A large proportion of long-standing detachments in any one series will probably contain a smaller percentage with tears. This partly accounts for the infrequency of such in certain series, viz. from 6·5 to 20 per cent. Other explanations may be incomplete dilatation of the pupil, opacities in the media, and varying knowledge of the diverse appearances assumed by openings in the retina. The peripheral position of the majority of tears, and the inability of some patients to rotate their eyes upwards, are other possible causes of discrepancies in the findings of tears in different series. Deutschmann (1926) found that tears were present in 17·4 per cent. of 539 detachments of the retina. He once considered all tears secondary, but now considers that some are primary. Schreiber found tears equally in myopes and non-myopes. In Nordenson's series of forty-five retinal tears, 50 per cent. were in the upper temporal area of the fundus; 25 per cent. in the lower half, and 2 per cent. in the lower nasal quadrant. Birch-Hirschfeld (1928) considers that a tear may be of considerable importance in producing a detachment of the retina, because he has found that spontaneously re-attached retinae showed no tear, and because those which did not heal usually showed one. He distinguishes primary from secondary tears, the latter being due to the dragging of the retina as the result of its shortening through glious growth of the retinal folds. Gonin (1928) has described one or more tears in fifty-three eyes in a series of sixty detachments; six of the remainder had opacities of the media which hindered examination. He stated that the majority occur in a narrow zone between ora serrata and equator, 7 mm. across, and so can be easily missed. Most other authors consider that tears vary in frequency, and that as a rule they are situated peripherally. Many observers considered that holes only appeared as secondary changes in a detachment of the retina, but the later series of Horstmann (1891 and 1898), with 45·7 per cent., and Gonin (1904–6), with at least 60 per cent. retinal tears, disprove this. These series showed that in nearly all detachments of the retina which had an abrupt onset, and were seen early, there was a tear. Later Leber reported twenty-three spontaneous detachments of the retina, of not more than two months' duration, in which a tear was found in all when first examined.

The size of the aperture found in detachment of the retina varies considerably. Nordenson (1887) published a series of forty-five detachments with tears, and of these, seven were very extensive, and yet not associated with injury. Leber referred to six similar tears, which were due to contusions. In Deutschmann's opinion very large tears are usually in the lower retina. Many of these large rents have sharp, jagged or shredded edges, in contrast with the round holes which are mainly due to cystoid degeneration. He considered that tears develop not only in those detachments which have a sudden onset, but also in slowly developing cases. One of his patients was a myopic teacher, blinded in the right eye by a detachment, whose left lower retina gradually became detached, showing three tears. After reaching a certain state it remained unchanged with good central vision for more than nine years. At times vessels are seen to bridge across a retinal rent. They may even be seen lying a considerable distance from the edges of the tear (Dunn, 1896; Doyne, 1902; Lacroix, 1919). Vogt (1930) has illustrated a large number of tears, showing their varied appearance. A number of his excellent illustrations are reproduced in Figs. 3 and 4, by his kind permission.

MACULAR HOLES. As the macula is the most delicate part of the retina, tears are not infrequent here. They are usually from one-third to one-half a disc diameter in width. Sometimes they are smaller, but Treacher Collins (1900) has described one equal in size to the papilla. They are usually round, sometimes slightly oval, and they appear clear cut as if cut out with a punching machine. The bared choroid shows clearly, and is dark red in colour. The surrounding retina is at first greyish white. Sometimes fine reflexes due to delicate folds radiate from a hole. Later little yellowish white spots appear on the base of the aperture, and the surrounding grey colour disappears. A difference in level, as a rule corresponding to from 1 to 1·5 D. (or $\frac{1}{3}$–$\frac{1}{2}$ mm.), and the presence of a parallax, clinch the diagnosis. If the hole is due to cystic degeneration, the remnants of cysts may be seen in the hole. Another point of distinction between these and the holes due to trauma is the presence of swelling round the hole in the latter, and its absence in the former (Vogt). Macular holes are best studied with red-free light. They appear to remain unchanged in appearance for long periods of time. In a patient reported by Harman (1901) a hole probably remained unchanged for forty-three years.

In 1869 Knapp described a macular hole for the first time. Two years later Noyes (1871) described one due to trauma. Little however was known of them, until Haab (1900) and Ogilvie (1900) discussed those due to trauma, and spontaneous holes were reported by Kuhnt (1900). Middleton's series (1919) is of interest. He collected it after the close investigation of 100,000 soldiers referred to a Special Medical Board in the United States Army. The twenty-three affected soldiers all gave a history of trauma, and one hole was associated with a detachment of the retina. Maxey (1918–19) reported three macular holes and one associated with detachment. Jackson reminds us that those which develop during later life may be due to myopic or vascular degeneration. Masuda (1919) refers to holes which followed an attack of iritis. Vogt (1924) reported a man with a retinal detachment, in which, during an attack of iritis, the sudden enlargement of a retinal tear was accompanied by acute hypotony. Macular holes may be due to a blow on the eye or to some other injury, or to retinal and choroidal inflammation of the anterior ocular tissues. They are found with chorio-retinitis (Pägenstecher, 1875; Zeeman, 1912), with retinitis pigmentosa (Nuel, 1896; Stock, 1908), and as a result of renal retinitis (Reis, 1906; and others). They may occur independently of other affections, and then are considered as primary. But usually some degree of vascular degeneration is present, and possibly a macular haemorrhage, which has been absorbed, may have caused the necessary damage to the tissue. Such cases have been described in middle-aged or younger patients by Küsel (1906), Zentmayer (1909), and Foster Moore (1910). Occasionally such a hole may be bilateral (de Schweinitz, 1904; Haab, 1908). Williamson (1921–2) considered that a macular hole could arise as a result of toxic influences. During irido-cyclitis toxins might act on the retinal veins causing thrombosis, and on the choroidal capillaries causing oedema. We owe much to Vogt (1925) and his followers for establishing, beyond doubt, as a clinical entity "cystoid macular degeneration" or honeycomb macula. Previously this condition was only known post-mortem (Fuchs, 1901, 1911; Coats, 1907). It is similar to cystoid degeneration (Iwanoff) in the retinal periphery. Vogt noticed it first in a young patient with retinitis pigmentosa. It is most frequently observed "in association with irido-cyclitis" (Vogt, 1925; Arnold, 1929). Especially when one is considering the cause of a detachment in the neighbourhood of the macula, it is well to remember this possibility.

Archangelsky (1925) has pointed out that the anatomical distribution of vessels in this area is particularly unfavourable to the resorption of fluid, and so a cyst may easily become a hole and lead to detachment. Differentiation may be difficult except in red-free light. Schieck (1929) considers that the posterior pole is most frequently and most extensively affected in metabolic and circulatory disorders, because this area is the most active physiologically, and therefore has the greatest metabolism. For this a large supply of serum is necessary, and as fewest vessels occur here, one may assume a greater permeability of the capillary endothelium. One can then imagine a greater leakage of serum and cells. Yellow-green light reveals in an unexpected manner the richness of the capillary system in the posterior pole.

Lister (1924) considers that a detachment of the retina with a peripheral hole is usually extensive, but that one associated with a macular hole is limited and non-progressive. Trauma and cystic degeneration may cause either variety. The holes may be hidden by folds in the detachment, or by vitreous opacities. In old detachments, tears often become invisible, therefore it is difficult to estimate their relative frequency. Lister cannot agree with Gonin that tears are always present. He considers that the variation in the nature of the inter-retinal fluid makes this unlikely.

Macular holes do not necessarily cause detachment of the retina, possibly because of surrounding adhesions. In fact Haab (1900) and later Lister, considered the association rare. E. von Hippel (1908), Leber (1916), Ellerhorst (1898), Dufour and Gonin (1906), Haab (1900), Dimmer (1898), Krusius, and many others, have described macular holes in detached retinae. Fleischer (1926) found a hole at each macula in a middle-aged patient with bilateral detachment of the retina.

There is a possibility that a macular hole may be secondary to the detachment. The following ways in which this may occur have been suggested:

1. The inter-retinal fluid may possess a tissue-injuring action.

2. Eye movements may tear this delicate area (Purtscher).

3. A shrinking vitreous or a preretinic membrane may tear an adherent retina from the choroid (Leber, von Hippel).

4. A tear may occur if some disorder develops in the intimate physiological relationship between the retina and the choroid (Hehr, 1920).

TRAUMATIC MACULAR HOLES. Noyes (1871), Dufour and Gonin (1906), Reis (1906), Purtscher (1909), von Szily (1919) and many recent observers have described trauma as a cause of macular holes. Salzmann (1919) found eight examples of macular holes due to war injuries among 2400 soldiers.

The commonest cause of a macular hole is a blow on the anterior part of the eye. If a tear of the posterior part of the retina does occur, it is nearly always at the macula. The structure and the situation of this part of the retina make it peculiarly susceptible to injuries of this kind. And tears near the posterior pole are usually here. Chevallereau's patient (1902) is exceptional. As a result of a blow from a large piece of wood, a tear 4 P.D. in length was found 2 P.D. from the optic disc. The edges were curved outwards, gradually separated and a detachment developed. Finnoff (1920) reported a macular hole with a separate rupture, half a disc diameter away.

PLATE III

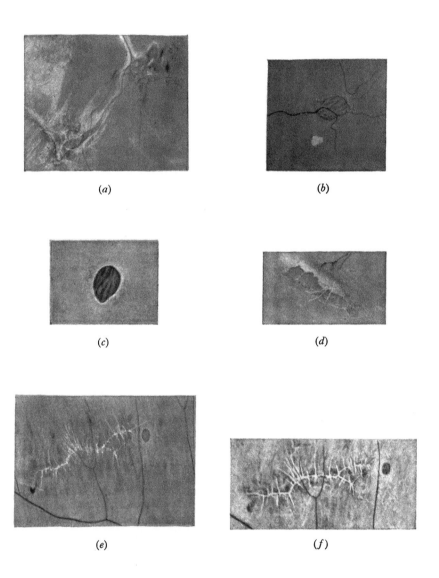

(a)

(b)

(c)

(d)

(e)

(f)

(a) A three-cornered tear, and below a group of folds with irregular cyst-like spaces. (b) A small hole. (c) A retinal hole, stamped out. (d) A retinal tear. (e) Striated white lines, with small holes. (f) The same fundus as (e) by red-free light.

(These illustrations are reproduced by kind permission of Professor Vogt and the publishers of the *Klin. Monatsbl. f. Augenheilk.*, F. Enke, of Stuttgart.)

The majority of macular holes can be traced to some preceding contusion. In the series of Haab and Ogilvie, only 3 out of 27 were considered due to other causes. In some cases there is a considerable interval after the injury before the hole appears (Holden, 1904; Haab, case 5, 1900; Twietmayer, case 1, 1907), whilst in other cases the hole was found on the day following the blow, or during the first week (Ogilvie's 7th case, 1900; Noll, 1908; Quint, 1906; Reis, 1906). Histological examination in Kipp's and Alt's (1908) and Coats's (1907) cases proved that trauma was the direct cause. In all eyes where a macular hole has directly followed injury, the force of the blow has been great. A thrown ball or stone, a flying piece of iron or wood, a shot arrow or bullet, or a blow from a fist or a stick, have caused most cases. Leber suggested that it was the area not supported by the capillary net in which the hole formed. The diameter of this is 0·4–0·5 mm. which corresponds with the usual diameter of a hole, namely 0·5 to 0·75 mm. The slight discrepancy he explained by the retraction of the edge. Red-free light demonstrates an individual variation in the non-vascular area. This may account for the variation in the diameter of macular holes. In the majority of cases, owing to its transient nature, Berlin's concussion change is not seen (Stähli, 1916; Purtscher, 1916).

Sometimes macular holes follow trauma indirectly. There is an interval during which some inflammatory or degenerative processes develop. This group is intermediate between the former group and the spontaneous "cases which follow degeneration". Leber considered that in infected injuries of the anterior ocular tissues a macular chorio-retinitis appeared. If later a detachment develops, the retina remains adherent to the choroid at this site. Investigations by Treacher Collins (1896) of this condition have been very illuminating. In other cases where cystoid degeneration was in existence at the time of injury, trauma plays the exciting part in producing the tear.

TRAUMATIC PERIPHERAL HOLES. A retinal tear following trauma is less common than a choroidal tear, mainly because the retina lies loosely on the pigment epithelium, whilst the choroid is firmly attached to the sclera by vessels and nerves. As the retina is most delicate near the periphery, tears are most frequent here. The peripheral tears may be rounded like the macular ones, but their shapes are diverse. They may be slit-like, angular, three-cornered, or horseshoe-shaped. The edges of the tears are usually turned inwards towards the vitreous, though Schweigger (1883) found the reverse condition to be more frequent.

Peripheral holes due to trauma are usually large. They are practically always associated with detachment. Exceptions are occasionally described (Lister, 1924). In such cases there are probably adhesions between the margins of the tear, and the choroid or vitreous, and the hole is virtually sealed.

The retina may be avulsed at the ora serrata, and its anterior edge turned down. In Scheffels' series (1890), one eye actually showed the external surface of the retina exposed to the observer's view through the pupil. This clearing away at the ora serrata may be due to shrinking bands in the vitreous due to haemorrhage or inflammation. As already described during discission a tearing away of the retina may occur if the "secondary cataract" has become connected to the retina close to the ciliary region. Fuchs (1877) described such an occurrence, in which the retinal dialysis was visible through the coloboma.

SPONTANEOUS PERIPHERAL LACERATIONS AND HOLES. Such apertures are nearly always found in association with detachment. It is known that independently of myopia, cysts and holes can develop as degenerative changes due to the influence of toxic spoiling and vascular lesions. Other theories have been put forward to account for them. Rählmann, for example, considered that the tension in the inter-retinal space, due to the diffusion of fluid through the retina, could become so great that a rupture would occur. This appears to be quite improbable. Elschnig considered that adhesions between the retina and choroid, due to a previous retino-choroiditis, could produce a tear if later a detachment did occur. Where holes in the retina are seen and

PLATE IV

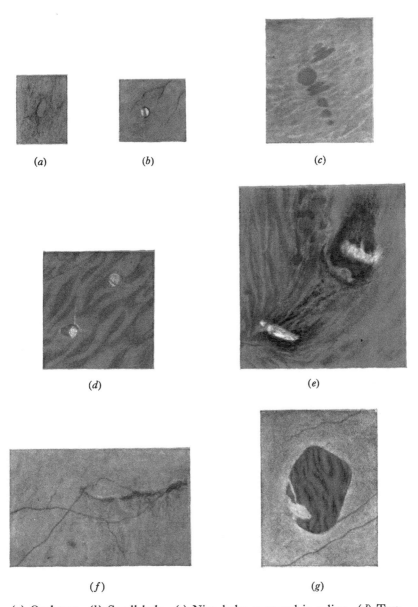

(a)   (b)   (c)

(d)   (e)

(f)   (g)

(a) Oval tear. (b) Small hole. (c) Nine holes arranged in a line. (d) Two small grey discs (lids) covering holes. (e) The retina of (d) after cautery puncture of both holes. (f) Split in retina. (g) Hole in senile retina.

(These illustrations are reproduced by kind permission of Professor Vogt and the publishers of the *Klin. Monatsbl. f. Augenheilk.*, F. Enke, of Stuttgart.)

a patch of degenerate retina is found adherent to the choroid in a corresponding position, this appears to be a suitable explanation. Lister refers to the incompleteness of the accounts of this condition. In Elschnig's first reported patient, a patch of retino-choroiditis was seen, and at a later examination a corresponding hole was found. The condition was not substantiated anatomically. In neither of Collins's patients was the retinal hole seen, though a patch of degenerated retina was found attached to the choroid. Rounded holes in the periphery are due to cystoid degeneration, and the adherence of a small disc to the choroid during detachment. Rarely does a disc become adherent to and detached into the vitreous, though Leber and Gonin describe instances. Leber and Nordenson explained these tears by postulating a previous vitreous haemorrhage or inflammation. Fibrous bands formed in the vitreous, and others united this body to the retina. Opacities in the media made ophthalmoscopic examination difficult. To support this explanation, there are macroscopic findings of a fibrinous effusion into the vitreous in plastic cyclitis which organises and contracts, and of vitreous bands causing wrinkling and detachment of the retina. Microphotographs by Lister (1924) show this clearly. If a retained foreign body is the cause of the retinal folds, the media may be clear and then they are seen most clearly by red-free light (Vogt, 1920, 1921).

Vogt states that probably in spontaneous detachments of the retina also a retinal tear is the cause. The aperture, he considers, is usually due to retinal degeneration. The actual detachment is probably precipitated by some slight trauma. Vogt does not deny the possibility of detachment of the retina without an aperture. However, he considers that, when tears are not seen, it is usually either because the detachment of the retina is old, with more or less opaque media, and an atrophic retina, or because they are situated in the extreme periphery. It appears almost certain that the majority of traumatic detachments are due to tears. As Vogt (1929) points out, the tear is usually in the periphery, because the retina is thinnest there, and less reinforced by the nerve-fibre layer. He considers that one can nearly always find a tear on the summit of the blister-like detachment. He has found a similar appearance in the majority of fresh non-traumatic or spontaneous cases. The tear often has jagged edges. Once formed it tends to increase in size, probably as the result of the movement of the body and of the eye. Vogt emphasises the fact that such an enlargement is favoured by the motion of the specifically heavier retina in the vitreous. To prove the greater specific gravity of the retina, he has centrifugalised small fragments of retina in vitreous. He finds in this also the explanation of the fact that tears of the upper retina are most usually associated with detachment. As a result of man's upright posture the relatively heavy retina, if degenerate, will yield first to any strain. Conversely, observations show that tears of the lower retina are least dangerous. Total detachment is most rare when the tear is situated in this area. Not only the greater specific gravity of the subretinal fluid but also that of the retina makes an upper detachment liable to become total.

SUDDEN DETACHMENT AND RETINAL HOLES. Leber has stated that sudden retinal detachment could not occur without a hole. Lister (1924), when recently supporting this idea, wisely emphasised the need to substantiate the history of a "sudden" onset. It may simply mean a sudden and belated discovery of a more or less long-standing visual loss. He stated, "With an intact eyeball and an intact retina, no detachment can take place unless there is a simultaneous and practically corresponding outpouring of fluid into the inter-retinal space on the one hand, and contraction of the vitreous on the other. Such pouring out of inter-retinal fluid and absorption of the vitreous, cannot of course take place suddenly. The onset of any detachment of the retina without a hole must therefore of necessity be gradual....It would therefore appear that if it can be substantiated, in any given case, that the loss of sight from detachment was not merely suddenly detected, but actually occurred suddenly, we can definitely predict the presence of a hole, whether or not it can be seen by the ophthalmoscope". It appears that this absolute statement "sudden onset—certain hole" must be modified. A peripheral detachment may be due to choroidal exudation, and no interference with vision be detected until it suddenly extends and becomes more central. Leber refers to shallow peripheral detachments which were undetected for a considerable time. Vogt repeats Schweigger's statement made years ago that peripheral tears and detachments may exist for a long time before the patient is aware of their presence. The possibility of this is shown by one of Lister's own patients. Here most certainly a rent was present, but the detachment, which was in the inferior periphery, remained stationary for at least four months. During this time vision was 6/6 and Jaeger 1, and the field was practically complete. If this can occur, retinal detachments, if peripheral, can remain undetected for some time if no tear is present. The aqueous may be squeezed out and space made for a sudden effusion. In this sense the eyeball may be regarded as being normally not "intact". Little is as yet known of the reaction of the vitreous to injury and toxins. Dehydration may occur which might enable a choroidal effusion to ensue. Certainly the development of the detachment and the tear do not always coincide. Lister refers to a medical student who received numerous blows about his head. It was not until eight days later, however, while climbing up the steps of an omnibus that the sight in one eye suddenly failed. When examined a large detachment with a large rent was found. Possibly some jerking movement or some sudden strain may be necessary to raise the retina from its normal position or force the vitreous through the hole. The younger the patient and the healthier the vitreous, the longer this may take. It may never occur if the margins of the tear unite to the retinal pigment epithelium. The vitreous, altered by trauma or toxic influences in this area, may seal the hole, as appears to be the case in experimentally produced detachments at times.

One can conclude that the majority of detachments which arise suddenly are associated with hole formation, but not that the relationship is essential and absolute.

THE THEORY OF ATTRACTION

As distension will not explain detachment of the retina in non-myopic eyes and eyes not affected by trauma, other theories must be considered. The theory of attraction will be considered second, because of its intimate relationship with the question of retinal tears, a subject already discussed. Müller (1858) found in many eyes that the vitreous contained much fibrous tissue, and was adherent to the retina. Such tissue was considered to be the cause of detachment of the retina in phthisis bulbi, in injured eyes, and in eyes where connective tissue followed intra-ocular inflammation or haemorrhage. Frequently the condition could not be diagnosed by the ophthalmoscope, and so this theory rested on the misleading histological evidence of eyes with long-standing detachment. Later this mechanism was forced to explain detachment of the retina in eyes free from injury or inflammation. This was largely the cause of its unpopularity. For opponents of this theory and possibly too ardent supporters emphasised the vitreous changes and referred to well-defined cords or membranes. Leber (1916) wrote, "The mention of such structures has been wrongly and repeatedly ascribed to me; neither ophthalmoscope nor microscope permitted one to recognise such changes". However, such changes sometimes do appear after vitreous haemorrhage and cause detachment (Gonin, 1920).

Leber (1882) noticed tears and detachment occurring together in eyes with retained foreign bodies. He introduced, aseptically, metallic bodies into the vitreous, and watched the formation of retinal tears, and after a few days extensive detachments of the retina. Rählmann (1893) detected similar changes after injecting a solution of sodium chloride into the vitreous. But here osmosis probably plays some part. Leber was impressed by the slightness of the force necessary to detach a retina in these experiments.

LEBER'S FIRST THEORY: *vitreous strands*. As a basis for the theory of attraction, Leber postulated the filling of the posterior part of the vitreous chamber with free fluid. Arlt's finding (1876) of such fluid in advanced myopia was amongst the original evidence which Leber collected to justify his attitude. He stated that this fluid was "free fluid which had collected on the inner retinal surface in consequence of vitreous degeneration". This, as will be seen, was also the evidence on which Iwanoff based his theory of vitreous detachment. Later Elschnig found vitreous liquefaction to be less common than Arlt considered it. He found it only four times in twenty-two myopic eyes. Leber found in this an explanation of the fact that not all myopes develop detachment of the retina. He stated further that in all cases of detachment of the retina investigated by him, he failed to find vitreous humour in the posterior part of the chamber; it being replaced by serous fluid which was usually separated sharply from the vitreous itself. In certain eyes the fluid completely replaced the humour.

Leber further considered that the sharp edges of the aperture suggested a tear due to traction, rather than a hole due to degeneration. He found that ophthalmoscopy failed to reveal any sign of degeneration near the aperture. As the rents were usually in front of the equator, he considered it unlikely that observers would see the strands or fine vitreous changes which produced the rents. He stated that the structure, which originates the "pull", acts in the region of the pars ciliaris, and so escapes direct observation. "It is noticeable almost solely through its consequences." If the retina is kept taut it will rupture when a certain tension is reached, and the free fluid will run through the tear and raise up the retina. Jerking eye movements might actually cause a tear. The photopsia seen before a detachment develops were considered to be due to the tugging on the retina by these strands. No increase in the tension of the eye was to be expected.

According to Leber's theory, epithelial cells proliferate from the ciliary body as a result of a slight inflammation of the pars plana of the ciliary body. They spread over the retina and into the vitreous. They become degenerate, and form fibrous bands which shrink and aid in the destruction of the solid vitreous—"fibrillary degeneration of the vitreous".

Contraction of these bands will cause a retinal tear, and later, when fluid passes through, retinal detachment occurs. Müller, de Wecker, Nordenson, and many others supported this view, and so the primary cause of spontaneous detachment of the retina was supposed to be an altered vitreous, which retracted the retina. This view is supported by the findings in retinitis proliferans.

Microscopic studies show a proliferation of epithelial cells in the vitreous, close to the ciliary body. If these cells become detached, they appear in the vitreous as floaters. Gonin says that they appear more lamellar or band-like than ordinary floaters. Other characteristics are their sudden appearance, and the lack of change in appearance over long periods of time. Fuchs (1923) has remarked that "since that surface of the ciliary body which looks backwards and inwards adjoins the vitreous, and is separated from it only by fibres of the zonula, it is easy to understand that in case of severe inflammation, leucocytes will pass from the ciliary body into the vitreous".

A similar mechanism, though in an exaggerated form, explains a rare form of detachment. Embryonic remains occasionally join the posterior surface of the lens or the ciliary region to the disc, and have been considered as factors in producing a detachment of the retina (Rollet and Rosnoblet, 1924; Lauber, 1924).

The difficulty in proving this theory has always been to show the necessary vitreous change which causes traction. Leber described a highly myopic eye which showed a fine fibrillary degeneration of the vitreous, adhesion of the latter to the retina, and fold formation of the retina due to the pull of a delicate bundle of fibrils. The folds were adherent to the vitreous by means of a tissue rich in cells. Nordenson (1887) soon afterwards supported him with findings from four enucleated eyes. Gonin (1904) reported findings in three eyes with spontaneous tears and detachments of the retina, and considered that in them no other plausible explanation was possible.

LEBER'S SECOND THEORY: "*preretinitis*". Later, in collaboration with von Hippel (1900 and 1908), Leber modified his views. For a long time he had noticed adhesions between the vitreous and the internal limiting membrane of the retina. These he considered were due to a preretinitis which formed an inflammatory membrane uniting the two structures. The shrinkage of this membrane was now considered the cause of the retinal tears. He described in great detail a condition which he called "primary retinal contraction". This is a wrinkling of the retina due to shrinkage of it and of the vitreous as a result of a hyalitis excited by retinal inflammation. This is in contradistinction to secondary retinal contraction, a condition obviously due to cyclitis or to any inflammation causing the formation of connective tissue in the vitreous, as seen typically in most cases of phthisis bulbi.

Leber believed that the new tissue due to the preretinitis probably arose from the pars ciliaris and the pigmented epithelium. Similar membranes have been demonstrated in myopic eyes. The vitreous change now assumed a more passive rôle, and was considered to be the result of a proliferation from this new tissue. As the new tissue contracted it raised the retina into folds, and fluid could collect underneath it, either through a retinal tear or as a transudation—"ex vacuo". (Such a theory makes cures rather hard to explain.) A fall in tension due to cyclitis or trauma, whether perforating or not, was emphasised as an important contributing factor. Leber distinguished a primary and exciting fall in tension from the usual secondary reduction.

GONIN'S MODIFICATION. Gonin (1923) has demonstrated by a series of histological examinations that in the periphery of the vitreous a migration of pigmented and unpigmented cells does occur, and that epithelial bands can produce traction on the retina, as can be seen at the edges of certain tears. He considers that as the bands are situated in front of the equator they are too far forwards to be seen by the slit-lamp. More recently he has stated that a band is insufficient to produce a detachment, unless it first causes a retinal tear. This may be due to the straining on adhesions during ocular movements or physical exertion. Recently, he has added as a factor adhesions of the retina and vitreous as a result of chorio-retinitis, which he finds of common occurrence in the equatorial zone.

Gonin differs from Leber by emphasising an equatorial choroiditis as the primary lesion, whilst Leber stressed "fibrillary degeneration" and later a shrinking preretinitic membrane. Gonin (1929) considers that, as a result of subsequent atrophy of the ciliary body, the epithelial cells proliferate from the uvea. He believes that retinal tears due to vitreous retraction are constant in spontaneous detachment of the retina. He stated that retinal cysts and tears may develop independently of the vitreous, but as a rule, adhesions to the vitreous predispose to their development. Heine (1924), after the microscopic examination of one hundred myopic eyes with retinal detachment, supported Gonin's views. He found that equatorial choroiditis was a frequent cause of myopic detachment of the retina. Gonin's theory postulates tears as primary and subretinal fluid as vitreous, in some form or other. It brings spontaneous detachments of the retina into line with those which follow haemorrhage into the vitreous, whether due to trauma or degeneration.

VITREOUS DETACHMENT. It is necessary to consider the mechanism that produces vitreous detachment, for it may throw light on the origin of retinal detachment. That vitreous bands occasionally play a part is undoubted. Fuchs describes two globes in which the anterior part of the retina and the ciliary body had been detached by shrinking membranes which followed trauma. Similar changes probably explain detachment of the retina after cataract extraction or discission. Just as the slit-lamp has proved that vitreous prolapse into the anterior chamber is an almost regular occurrence after needling a secondary cataract (Comberg, 1924; Erggelet, 1914; and others), so it can reveal strands running posteriorly. Meisner (1925) reports an incident worthy of mention. No vitreous was lost at the time of operation, and no post-operative infection occurred, and yet a cord of "thickened vitreous" was found to run from the discission scar through the vitreous to the site of the detachment (Sinclair, 1916; Roberts, 1919). Ralston and Goar (1922), Basterra Santa-Cruz (1924), and Ringle (1923), amongst others, have reported one or more detachments after cataract operations. (NOTE. It appears that retinal detachments are considerably more frequent after discission than after extraction, and that injury to the vitreous must be avoided at all costs.) If traction plays the main part in the production of a detachment of the vitreous, a retinal detachment may occur, if the two structures are adherent. The vitreous never becomes detached in the neighbourhood of the ciliary body, because of its firm attachment there (Fuchs, 1923). If traction can cause either form of detachment, this attachment may be one factor which makes this area specially susceptible to retinal detachment. Pillat (1922, 1925) and Lister (1922) have shown the part played by fibrous bands, either congenital or acquired, in producing a detachment of the vitreous. Injury, haemorrhage or inflammation lead to the adhesion of the vitreous to the internal limiting membrane. Sudden movement or prolonged strain or contraction of vitreous bands may cause detachment of the vitreous, or even of the retina. A bullous, annular or funnel-shaped vitreous detachment may be formed. A hole may show on the surface of the vitreous. Occasionally a hole has been described in "the hyaloid membrane". The adherence of the vitreous to the entrance of the optic nerve when the former shrinks away from the retina would account for central holes. Kraupa (1923, 1924, 1925), Isakowitz (1926), Rea (1923) and Gimblett (1923) each describe this condition. In the fundus described by Goldstein (1923) an almost circular hole was seen, and a patch of chorio-retinal atrophy of corresponding size. Purtscher's patient (1919) showed a similar appearance. Kraupa has seen tears in the periphery of the vitreous with an arc-lamp. Vitreous detachment is a condition probably not always recognised because of the vitreous opacities accompanying it.

Iwanoff (1869) was the first to explain the association of detachment of the retina and advanced myopia by considering that a detachment of the vitreous was an essential factor. He believed that the liquefied posterior vitreous segment was in reality a collection of fluid between the vitreous and the retina. More extensive anatomical investigations by Leber, de Wecker, and Elschnig have shown that this can be only an exceptional occurrence. De Wecker considered that as the fluid in the vitreous increased, the retina was torn, and fluid passed under the retina and so produced detachment, whilst Leber considered the tears were due to the traction of newly formed tissue in the vitreous.

CRITICISM OF TRACTION THEORY. Hanssen (1919) and Vogt (1924) consider that the epithelial proliferation described by Gonin is rarely, if ever, primary. They agree that the cystoid degeneration, so common near the ora serrata in myopes, and senility are the main conditions necessary for a tear; trauma only playing a part by forcing degenerate vitreous through the aperture and raising up the retina. Vogt (1923) considers Leber's theory unlikely, because he has never observed with slit-lamp or ophthalmoscope any vitreous bands in a recent detachment of the retina, or in an eye prior to the development of a detachment. Koby (1925) has not found vitreous bands in myopic eyes which could be considered instrumental in causing a retinal detachment. But Comberg (1924) says that very delicate vitreous strands can be seen in some cases of ocular injury by the slit-lamp only, and that possibly these may take part in the production of a detachment of the retina.

Fuchs (1920) considers it quite probable that in the eyes with detachment of the retina due to traction, other changes in the form of opacities may be sufficient to hide the bands ophthalmoscopically. One must remember however that in Leber's experiments the vitreous remained clear even though strands did exist and produce detachments.

Vogt finds the structure of the myopic vitreous very defective. He considers that the more solid masses in the vitreous, "Glaskörperbasis" (Salzmann), may cause the downward pull necessary for a detachment of the retina. They are most numerous in the periphery near the ora serrata. To these the framework of the myopic or senile vitreous adheres, and coils projecting from the vitreous unite it to the retina. These coils move more rapidly than normal vitreous if the eye moves. By these traction can be exerted on the retina. The vitreous framework, as described by Vogt, is degenerative, and not inflammatory or cicatricial as conceived by Leber. Therefore it is difficult to account for detachment, especially in myopic eyes, by vitreous strands and "preretinitis". In extreme myopia it is unlikely that they play a part, because the vitreous is liquefied, and free from any fibrous strands. The shrunken vitreous, altered by a considerable change in pH, is not the kind of substance with which we would associate traction. Strand formation is not found with such dehydration. As already pointed out, the vitreous itself cannot form connective tissue strands. It requires a fibroblastic invasion from the mesoblast of the retinal vessels. The proliferated epithelial cells in the ciliary region, as described by Gonin, may conceivably degenerate into bands capable of traction, but it is not probable. It is also difficult to conceive of cure and re-attachment being possible if such a shrunken vitreous had actually caused the detachment.

Vogt considers it difficult to explain the characteristic change in position from upper to lower pole if the upper part of the retina is detached by traction downwards. It is equally difficult to understand the subsequent spontaneous re-attachment above, if this theory holds. If they pull downwards in the initial stage, they are not likely to pull in a different direction later. As Hanssen (1919) suggests, if the traction factor was as important as Gonin and others assure us it is, detachment would be observed earlier, and more frequently in retinitis proliferans. Deutschmann (1928-9) does not agree with Gonin that tears are usually causative in myopia. He thinks that if they were, the inter-retinal fluid would be the same clinically as vitreous. His observations that at times tears heal, and detachments persist, and that incisions made by him in the ora serrata led to tears which healed and yet left the detachment unchanged, support his antagonism. In his experiments, and clinically, Weekers (1925) found tears in the retina over the fluid which collects under the secondary detachment in the lower pole. These he

considered due to degeneration. He considers that a detachment of the retina can occur without the slightest tear.
"Ces déchirures sont un accident: elles sont loin d'être
constantes." They are independent of the state of the
vitreous, and are the result of sudden effusion from the
choroid. This area of the retina gradually degenerates, but
the underlying exudate persists. The retina becomes folded,
producing an appearance of cyst formation, due to consequent disturbances in circulation. Weekers considers that
certain authors (Iwanoff) considered these to be true cysts,
and even the cause of detachment of the retina. Hanssen
(1915) reported that histological examination of both eyes of
a patient with spontaneous detachment of the retina failed to
reveal any sign of bands in the vitreous, or any cellular
membranes on the inner retinal surface, or ciliary hyper-
plasia. The patient had numerous ocular operations, including a cataract extraction. He (1919) gives the histological
findings in two eyes in which membranes were found present
on the inner retinal surface. The details were entirely
different from those characteristic of idiopathic detachment
of the retina. He considers that the evidence for the theory
of attraction is based on the findings in old detachments. He
adds that it is unlikely that connective tissue membranes
should arise from ciliary epithelium. Both Hanssen and
Vogt have frequently found membranes on both sides of the
degenerate retina. Therefore they consider the bands, that
Gonin considers primary, to be secondary. The presence of
subretinal cellular and fibrous formations in old cases
suggests that such tissue is the result of detachment of the
retina rather than a cause.

Fuchs (1921) has described a series of globes in which the
retinal and disc vessels were dragged from their normal
position by shrinking retinal scars and exudates. They
showed little or no tendency to detachment of the retina, even
though in four of them the dragging was due to membranes
at the anterior margin of the retina. Cyclitic membranes had
drawn each anterior margin forwards about 3·5 mm., and
each disc appeared distorted. In one eye the retina was so
pulled forwards that, posteriorly, it covered the temporal

half of the disc, and anteriorly it was adherent to the posterior lens surface. He describes a similar forward displacement of the anterior margin in the senium due to condensation of the vitreous in the anterior part, and its pull on the retina.

THE THEORY OF DEPRESSION

A sudden loss of vitreous or a gradual atrophy of the eye may cause a detachment by the withdrawal of the force which normally assists in keeping the retina in position. This is the reverse state to that described as "distension".

THE HYDROSTATIC THEORY. Baurmann (1928–9) has expressed the view that many detachments are due to an upset of the hydrostatic equilibrium. He considers that to fulfil its function, viz. the nourishing of the deep retinal layers, the choroid must maintain a certain minimum volume of blood flowing through its capillaries. For the circulation of fluid through the tissues, he considers the following driving forces: (a) the hydrostatic pressures in the tissues, and in the blood track; (b) the osmotic pressure. Baurmann considers that detachments are due to a disturbance of the equilibrium of the pressure on each side of the retina. An exudative choroiditis is the commonest cause of such a disturbance. He believes that tears are only secondary, but that they are a hindrance to re-attachment.

If the inter-retinal space has a lower capillary pressure than the preretinal space, a resorption excess occurs, and the former space is reduced to a latent cleft. If, however, the inter-retinal capillary pressure rises above the preretinal capillary pressure, there is an exit of protein from the choroidal vessels, causing a detachment, and finally the retina will become torn. As soon as a rent occurs there will be equalisation of pressure on the two sides of the retina. So, as Lister suggests, only one hole can be produced by pressure on the outer retinal surface. If a sudden drop in the pre-retinal capillary pressure occurs or if the walls of the choroidal capillaries become more permeable to proteins, the retro-retinal colloidal osmotic pressure will exceed that in the preretinal space, and a detachment will develop. He considers that extensive destruction of the chorio-capillaris a probable cause of raised capillary pressure. There being few capillaries to carry the minimum essential volume of blood, the pressure must rise. Choroidal degeneration or vitreous loss could cause the necessary reduction in the preretinal pressure.

When we come to consider the results of Gonin's method of treatment, it will be of value to recall this theory. By his results, the ease with which the retina returns to and adheres in its old position is demonstrated. The subretinal fluid, too, promptly disappears, and does not return once the hole is closed. This suggests that the normal excess of preretinal pressure is restored. The vitreous turgescence presses the retina back into position, and enables a restoration of the intimate relations of the visual elements and the pigment epithelium to occur. The integrity of the retina is essential if this excess pressure, delicate though it be, is to maintain this relationship on which vision depends.

It is quite probable that in the myope the available amount of normal vitreous and consequently the turgescence is reduced. After trauma slit-lamp microscopy reveals delicate fibrils in the vitreous. If these are associated with dehydration, possibly not only in the myopic but also in injured eyes will the vitreous be less able to press towards the choroid.

Baurmann's histological report on the eye of a patient with glaucoma is of interest. On doing the iridectomy during a trephine operation, vitreous was lost. Three days later an extensive detachment was visible. Neither a shrinking vitreous nor a contracting band, but only an effusion behind the retina could explain this. Histologically a markedly albuminous fluid was present. Anteriorly a tear was found, and glious membranes stretched from it to the vitreous, lens and iris. He considered that the choroid capillaries had become more permeable to protein bodies by the sudden removal of pressure. With that the effective colloid osmotic pressure of the serum had fallen, while the double epithelium covering the ciliary vessels prevented the passage of protein. As the intra-ocular pressure was reduced, fluid had to be exuded from the choroid as soon as the effective colloid osmotic pressure became lower than the choroid capillary pressure.

De Decker (1929) found in his series of detachments of the retina of unknown origin that a capillary upset was present in 25 per cent. There was in these cases an increase in intra-ocular pressure of the affected eye during the "period of blood plasma increase". Whereas in normal eyes the intravenous saline injection did not alter intra-ocular pressure, it caused a rise during the blood plasma increase in the affected eye of those with detachment. Results with the drinking test were similar.

Baurmann described also the eyes of a myope (14–16 D.). There was scattered lymphocytic infiltration of the choroid and a marked atrophy of the chorio-capillaris. Fluid with a high protein content was found under each retina. In one eye several tears were found which were closed by a firmly attached vitreous. Delicate vitreous membranes were present. Baurmann considered that, as a result of atrophic choroidal vessels, protein could escape, and so the normal resorption excess of the inter-retinal space was altered to a resorption deficiency. He explained a partial re-application of the detachment to a late restoration of the normal relation of pre-retinal and inter-retinal pressures. The partial fixation by the membranes prevented complete re-application. On the basis of measurements of the protein content of the inter-retinal fluid, it is to be assumed that the inter-retinal protein gradually loses its colloid osmotic effectiveness by the aggregation of its particles. This upset in the hydrostatic balance may explain certain detachments. If a detachment is not due to tumour formation, or haemorrhage, or inflammation, Baurmann's theory may be applicable. The low tension in these cases is not comparable in effect with the markedly reduced tension in general disorders, e.g. diabetic coma, or severe diarrhoea or cholera. The general dehydration reduces the tension, but detachment has not been observed.

THE INCIDENCE OF LOW TENSION. Baurmann (1924) considers that no subretinal fluid can collect unless tension is reduced. When tension falls, fluid can be given off by the vascular

chorio-capillaris. Halbertsma (1926) has found exceptionally
low tension as an early sign of detachment of the retina in
myopia. Gallois (1927), Gonin (1920), and many others have
also written on this association with hypotony. It is interesting to compare this finding with those cases of detachment
which have improved when an attack of glaucoma super-
vened (Sedan, 1928). Axenfeld, Baurmann and Vogt have
observed the tension fall in primarily glaucomatous eyes
when a detachment has occurred. Thomas (1925), in a series
of 247 affected patients in the Kiel Clinic from 1913 to 1924,
found only one with raised tension. In some, the detachment
of the retina followed prolonged hypotony. He considers it
difficult to understand why fluid does not re-absorb if
tension is normal. Kümmell (1919, 1921) reported forty-two
cases of hypotony in fifty-two eyes with detachment of the
retina, and he concluded that an affection of the ciliary
process produced this hypotony, and the accompanying
vitreous degeneration, and caused a choroidal transudation.
Fuchs (1923) considers that in low-grade myopia the detachment of the retina is due to low tension, and that it may
be preceded by a detached vitreous. The cause of almost
inevitable recurrence lies in the fact that no treatment is able
to do away with the condition which usually lies at the
bottom of the trouble, viz. the altered state of the vitreous.
He states that intra-ocular pressure is generally reduced as a
result of reduced volume of vitreous. For the same reason
the anterior chamber is deep, the lens having sunk backwards.

THE CAUSES OF LOW TENSION. Let us very briefly consider
the causes of low tension. Some are well known, and the
mechanism at work simple, but others are rare and abstruse.
The hypotony following perforation, whether it be from
trauma, ulceration, or operative interference, and that which
follows tight bandaging, require no comment. But the fall in
tension following corneal inflammation and slight injuries
is more difficult to understand. It suggests some nervous
mechanism. That such may be the case is supported by the
fall which follows paralysis of the sympathetic and the
experimental findings of Weekers (1924) and Leplat (1924).

Destructive lesions of the ciliary body from toxic influence or from trauma can produce low tension. Phthisis bulbi may follow these, or the shrinking of exudates in the vitreous which reduce its volume. The reaction of the vitreous to alterations in pH and osmotic pressure, in diabetes and other conditions where the blood composition is changed, is still indefinite.

Leber in his theory described a fibrillary degeneration of the vitreous. Disease of the choroid and of the ciliary body may produce a shrinking of the vitreous, so that it becomes detached from the retina, except at the disc and the ora serrata. In such a state a considerable proportion of the vitreous is replaced by fluid. This fluid can easily be displaced. Trauma can force aqueous out through Schlemm's canal, and displace the fluid of the vitreous forwards, and so remove the support from the retina in a different way. Beigelman (1929) describes what he considers a definite entity, viz. a detachment due to a sudden absorption of fluid vitreous, a subsequent acute lowering of tension, associated with a deepening of the anterior chamber, and a mild uveitis. Schnabel (1876) was the first to describe acute hypotony in retinal detachment. He considered it to be due to the bursting of a myopic staphyloma. Leber (1916) was the first to establish the association as a clinical entity. Lauber (1908) and Vogt (1924) considered that hypofunction of the ciliary body due to cyclitis caused the low tension. But Leber stated that a reduced formation of aqueous would be balanced by a reduced outflow and so tension would scarcely be affected. Beigelman considers that a sudden absorption of fluid from the vitreous by the chorio-capillaris through a retinal hole is the cause. This may be so, but it will not explain the collapsed eyeball of diabetic coma which will be considered shortly. The possibility of a rare condition such as "essential phthisis", ophthalmomalacia, producing a detachment is of interest. According to Fuchs, the eye suddenly becomes softened, smaller and injected. After several hours or days, the attack passes, but recurrences are not uncommon. Beigelman quotes Meller (1928) who wrote "the function of the epithelial cells of the ciliary body, and probably also of the retina, and the ora serrata, is absorption of fluid from vitreous, and its transmission along lymph channels". That this is possible is further suggested by Magitot's theory (1929). He states that the aqueous is formed by that which represents the pia mater and the nervous parenchyma, *i.e.* the uvea, principally the iris and the retina. The ocular liquid dialysed by the capillaries is absorbed by the same route. Normally there is no circulation of fluid in the true sense of the term. The exit and entrance of the liquid are two phenomena which balance each other, and are dependent on the nutritive demands of the nerve cells. He considers that the ciliary body, the structure of which is not particularly adapted for dialysis, possesses merely a dynamic rôle in vision (accommodation).

The degenerate condition of the vitreous, with the settling down of the more solid vitreous to the inferior pole, may account for the superior pole being the commonest site for the origin of detachment of the retina. The extreme importance of a normal vitreous is demonstrated in the detachments associated with the toxaemias of pregnancy. Even though the detachment is very extensive, it will almost certainly clear up completely. This is probably mainly due to a healthy vitreous. Detachment of the retina occurred in 1·2 per cent. of 1024 obstetric patients, an unusual number of whom were difficult cases, and in 10·4 per cent. of those with eclampsia (Fry, 1929). It is usually bilateral and most common at term. Killick (1921) stated that with a healthy vitreous, no detachment of the retina would exist. Meller considers that, even if no opacities be visible, the vitreous in detachment of the retina is always degenerate and usually liquid. However, not all eyes with fluid vitreous develop detachment of the retina, so other factors are necessary. It is difficult to decide whether this other factor is reduction of tension, traction by vitreous strands or hole formation, or subretinal effusion, as low tension is so frequently associated with retinal detachment that its influence must be considered.

THE EFFECTS OF LOW TENSION. The changes in the eye during a sudden and marked or a long-standing hypotony must be considered. Not only is there a sucking in of the inelastic cornea in old age, and a certain shrinking of the cornea in youth as the pressure in the anterior chamber falls towards the level of atmospheric pressure, but there is also a compression of the eye by the recti muscles, producing the typical bale-shaped appearance. These muscles also tend to retract and so force the globe against the contents of the orbit. This is apt, especially in myopia, to lead to a dimpling or reverse staphyloma of short duration after a cataract extraction (Fuchs, 1930). In hypotony, the lens, if present, will move forwards or backwards according to whether aqueous or vitreous has been lost. There will be a shrinking of the choroid and the sclera which the less elastic and normally less stretched retina cannot take part in. Therefore it will be raised into folds.

Two other changes take place. They are due to the upset in the normal balance of pressure. The first depends on a reversal of the relationship between intra-ocular pressure and intracranial pressure. To ensure the escape of lymph from the eye the former is normally the higher. When, however, it falls to the level of atmospheric pressure this lymph cannot escape, and so a mild papilloedema will develop, which can obscure a glaucomatous cup. Usually when papilloedema develops, conditions are the reverse. Probably when oedema of the disc, or a subhyaloid haemorrhage develops during a subarachnoid haemorrhage, the greatly increased pressure either forces blood and cerebro-spinal fluid along the lymph channels, or leads to diapedesis by restricting the retinal vein and lymphatics.

DETACHMENT OF THE CHOROID (v. Plate V a). The second change is due to the reduction of the intra-ocular pressure below the choroidal capillary pressure. Normally they are balanced, or only sufficient difference exists to enable an interchange of fluid. If the pressure in the choroidal capillaries is relatively increased, hyperaemia and a sucking out from them of serum, or actually of blood, may occur. If the latter, a secondary glaucoma may develop, which is essentially resistant to operative measures. If a serous transudation develops, a detachment of the choroid may ensue. Such a detachment appears as a smooth opaque and dark projection "which does not make undulating movements like a detached retina, and over which the retinal vessels pass without tortuosity" (Fuchs). It is transient in nature and the temporal or nasal peripheral portion is the most frequently affected. It rarely develops above or below, and never in the posterior pole. As Fuchs states, it can most easily be observed if after a trephine there is delayed formation of the anterior chamber. As a rule opacities in the media obscure such a detachment when it develops after perforating ulcers or injuries.

To show the relatively frequent occurrence of detachment of the choroid, Elliot (1922) quotes Meller who found it in 22 per cent. of eyes after Lagrange's operation, and Fuchs who found it in 4 per cent. after cataract extractions and 10 per cent. after glaucoma iridectomies.

One must ask why in such conditions does a detached choroid and not a detached retina result? Fuchs states that he has never seen a retinal detachment follow the loss of aqueous or vitreous, even though the eye collapses. Neither does it follow vitreous aspiration as practised by zur Nedden (1923). The choroid is more contractile than the sclera, especially in old age, and so it tends to become detached as a negative pressure is formed between them. In youth the sclera is more contractile, and it can be indented with ease in hypotony. Fuchs considers that greater resistance to separation is offered by two smooth moist surfaces such as those of the retina and the choroid, which at least are in intimate contact, than by the choroid and the sclera which are attached by most delicate lamellae. If, however, normal vitreous escapes, the retina is most likely to become detached because of its attachment to the vitreous near the ora serrata. Such a development follows a perforating injury rather than an operation.

The theory of exudation brings many cases of detachment of the retina into line with detachment of the choroid, in that the latter condition, as Fuchs and Kalt (1924) agree, is due to a transudation from a choroid with vascular degeneration.

PLATE V

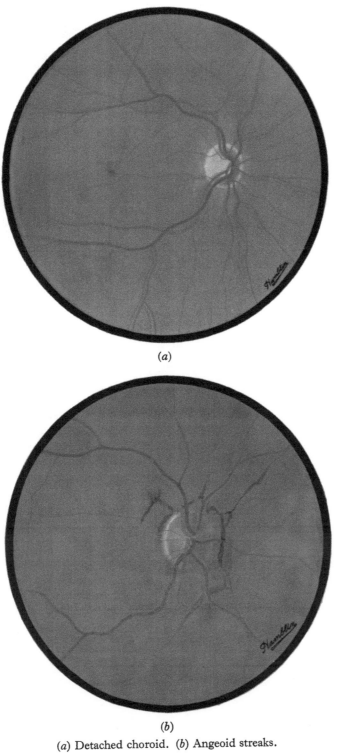

(a)

(b)

(a) Detached choroid. (b) Angeoid streaks.

E. Fuchs (1921) considers that the serous effusion comes from the capillaries and smallest veins. The sudden decrease in intra-ocular pressure is the main cause. Detachment of the choroid tends to clear up spontaneously. The good prognosis is associated with the fact that the fluid which collects does not descend, but remains at the site of the lesion where it can be most easily absorbed. It is possible that at times angioid streaks (*v.* Plate V *b*) are left behind, just as a re-attached retinal detachment may leave the appearance referred to as "retinitis striata" (Plocher, 1917; Guist, 1921).

Frank's remarkable case, which he had watched for five years (1921), convinced him of the influence that the choroid can have in exceptional cases. A bullous or folded detachment of the retina appeared and disappeared in angiomatosis. After histological examination it seemed that the detachment was due to vascular disturbance in the choroid, and that a temporary compensation of this could lead to re-attachment.

HYPOTONY IN DIABETIC COMA. The hypotony occurring in diabetic coma is very marked. With it one might expect retinal detachment to develop, but I have been unable to find a single case in the literature. It is interesting to note, however, that one choroidal detachment has been reported, which was probably due to dysentery (Verhoeff and Waite, 1925). This is not because the eyes of comatose patients have not been examined. The fall in tension is due to the content of salt and sugar in the ocular fluids (Patek, 1929). "The severe diabetic during coma utilizes apparently all possible liquid in the tissues to aid in the excretion of toxic bodies" (Joslin, 1928). Hypotony appears in coma for the same reason as a pre-existing oedema will disappear and the weight of the patient falls. "Oedema is as common an occurrence in the use of insulin as it is uncommon in coma." The oedema of insulin therapy may explain the retinal detachments which occur after its use at times. Alperin (1929) and McBean (1928) have described detachments following insulin therapy in four patients. In hypoglycaemia a greater amount of exudate, diffusate or transudate would be thrown out into the inter-retinal space because the normal equilibrium between the intra-ocular pressure and the capillary pressure is upset. Normally the intra-ocular pressure is lower than the capillary pressure, and so the fluid changes, necessary for metabolism, can occur. If a diabetic patient takes too much exercise one day (and a certain patient described a round of golf as the equivalent of five units of insulin), or if the patient eats too little, but still takes the amount of insulin prescribed for an average day, the hormone is free to act on the blood sugar, and hypoglycaemia may result. This means an elevation of the osmotic pressure of the blood because, as a result of the thinning of the blood, or in other words, the diluting of the electrolytes, the ionisation of the mineral salts will be greater. This increase in osmotic pressure, according to Alperin, can either produce its main ocular effect on the ciliary or on the choroidal blood systems. If the former, the ciliary processes become distended, and glaucoma results. If the latter, there may be an effusion under the retina and its subsequent detachment. In Richter's experiments (1926) glaucoma followed the administration of insulin. Marx (1925) also found that in three of five patients on insulin therapy, the intra-ocular pressure rose.

It is difficult to understand Vestergaard's results (1929). After the intravenous injection of insulin, he detected a fall in tension which lasted for an hour. A similar effect on tension follows the intravenous injection of epinephrine and hypophysin. Insulin lowers the blood sugar by aiding its conversion into a substance which can be stored in muscles and the liver, viz. glycogen. Insulin does not lessen the blood sugar by burning it, but by preparing and storing it for the tissues to burn. Insulin and a marked increase of carbohydrate in the diet promote the storage of glycogen in the liver and muscles, and oedema follows. This oedema is increased by the presence of diseased kidneys, for then the excretion of salt is defective. The acute myopia and the oedematous disturbance of the posterior layers of the iris in diabetes probably owe their origin to such an oedema. This emphasises the part that oedema may play, and the absence of detachment in the hypotony of coma shows the ineffectiveness of low tension when due to general dehydration. The dramatic rise in tension in a comatose patient after transfusion was first related to me by Dr Ewen Downie.

It is wise to consider briefly the cause of this low tension in coma. It was first described by Krause (1904), and later emphasised by Reisman (1916). In Joslin's clinic, in a series of fifty patients in whom tension was specially observed, it was found low in twenty-nine. He uses it as a diagnostic sign in the differentiation of hyperglycaemic coma or the coma of diabetic acidosis from hypoglycaemic coma, and that of nitrogen retention, whether due to nephritis, the toxic effects of infections and drugs, or to other causes. Other characteristics of diabetic coma, useful in the differentiation and of interest here, are the raised blood sugar content, and the reduced plasma CO_2 combining power. There is also a reduction of the pH of the blood. The value for oxalated blood may fall to pH 7·03 (normal 7·35). It is difficult to say how great a part this plays in reducing the ocular tension. The feel of the eyeball suggests a very definitely altered vitreous. A similar reduction in tension has been noted in Asiatic cholera and the severe diarrhoeas. Here, no doubt, the dehydration is due to other causes. Giffo (1924), Hertel (1915), Ascher (1925), Gallus (1924), Middleton (1923), Heine (1906), in referring to the low tension in diabetic coma, state that there is no corresponding fall in blood pressure. Joslin reaffirms this statement, though at times blood pressure does fall in coma.

The association of detachment with renal retinitis, and the absence of such with retinitis in diabetes, is worthy of note. The deciding factor in the former is probably the tendency to oedema. It is still a moot point whether a typical diabetic retinitis occurs. Of 307 diabetic patients 207 had normal retinae, and of these 98 per cent. had normal renal function, and 91 per cent. normal blood pressure. Every case of retinitis showed retinal arterio-sclerosis. By X-ray examination of the vessels in the lower extremities, 63 per cent. of patients over forty years of age were found to have arteriosclerosis, whilst only 28 per cent. of non-diabetic patients showed these changes (Bowen and Koenig, 1927). "The longer the duration of the diabetes, the greater the degree of arterio-sclerosis, and in the old the less severe the diabetes"

(Joslin, 1928, p. 173). The age incidence of diabetic retinitis corresponds with this statement. It is rarely if ever seen before thirty-five (Foster Moore). It seems that a characteristic retinitis appears in diabetes only when complicated by arterio-sclerosis (Wagener and Wilder, 1921). The importance of arterio-sclerosis in diabetes is further demonstrated by Joslin's finding that it is the cause of death in 47 per cent. of cases, and coma in only 20 per cent., whilst in the pre-Banting era, the figures were 15 per cent. and 61 per cent. respectively.

TRANSUDATE OR INFLAMMATORY EXUDATE. To establish the basis for this theory we must consider the question, " Is the choroidal lesion non-inflammatory and the fluid a transudate, or is it inflammatory with an exudation?" That it is often the former is the view of Kümmell (1924) who considers that a transudation is more probable than an inflammatory exudation. It is due to the marked hyperaemia of the vascular plexus which constitutes the choroid, when there is a steadily diminishing ocular tension. The hypotony frequently noted early in detachment of the retina strengthens this view. Kümmell (1921) reported forty-two eyes with low tension in a series of fifty-two detachments. Sixteen of these were of only two weeks' duration. He found the angle of the anterior chamber widely open, but in some cases pigmented material blocked the entrance to Schlemm's canal. Other signs of irido-cyclitis were present. He believed (1925 a) that low tension usually precedes detachment of the retina. Low tension due to retinal and choroidal degeneration and a shrinking vitreous produce a suction on the uveal vessels and a transudate results. Any difference in tension on the two sides of a degenerate retina could easily produce a tear.

Weekers (1924) quotes Hortsmann's series of 106 detachments, of which 46 had low tension, and 60 normal tension. Usually at the beginning the tension is normal. Only after several days or weeks does it become reduced. Weekers holds that if examined in an early enough stage, tension will be found raised. This early rise in tension being of short duration could easily escape notice. Schnabel and Samelsohn, however, stated that low tension actually precedes detachment of the retina. Leber considered that the fact that tension does not rise at the moment of detachment was proof that exudate did not cause detachment of the retina. Experimentally, however, immediately after cauterisation there is a sudden sharp short rise of tension, lasting four or five hours, followed by a prolonged fall. As shown later, the rise is due to the sudden exudate, and the fall probably to an excessive elimination of aqueous.

There are many detachments which have followed physical strain and hyperaemia of the head. Transudation is a possible explanation of these. Further light can be thrown on this question by a consideration of the effect of the marked vascular disturbance in the choroid following enucleation or death. There is a marked fall in blood pressure, and a shrinkage of the choroid. The consequent disproportion between the retina and the choroid leads to the formation of retinal folds. If the eye is removed after death no fluid will be found between the folds and the choroid. It is well known, however, that a thick fluid or jelly is present if the eye is removed during life. The extent of these folds, especially in the macular area, is very considerable.

Unfortunately histological examination of early detachments is rarely possible. Gonin, in reviewing the literature, stated that there was not one report of an examination of an eye with idiopathic detachment of the retina made when the conditions were fresh. Since then Kümmell (1928) examined histologically an eye with a detachment only seven days old. The only vitreous changes were unimportant. Two retinal tears were present. They were considered to have been in existence long before the detachment of the retina. Marked cystoid degenerative changes were found in the retina, with slight proliferation of the pigment epithelium. In part the retina was almost completely replaced by strands of connective tissue. The cystoid degeneration was most marked close to the tears; but, as he did not find such changes in other detached retinae, he is inclined to explain this detachment by the hydrostatic theory of Baurmann, and not by the cystoid degeneration theory of Hanssen and Gonin. The choroid and ciliary body were filled with blood. At some places the vessels were distended and arranged in knots. The other eye was practically normal. Kümmell considered that, to equalise the hypotony that existed, a sucking of the retina from the vitreous occurred, and simultaneously, as a result of the fall in pressure, a transudation set in from the overfull choroidal vessels, which pushed the retina before it. Other detachments with low tension reported by Kümmell (1925) are of interest. He considered that a steadily diminishing tension in the vitreous cavity could produce marked uveal hyperaemia and subsequent transudation. The following history he considers typical of a group of spontaneous detachments with low tension. The eye was moderately myopic. Dulling of the vitreous had been observed and the slit-lamp showed isolated floaters, not the thickened strands of Leber. Some months later a detachment of the retina suddenly developed, and hypotony was found. On account of uveitis, the eye was excised seven weeks later. The exact microscopic result revealed, as the most important fact, the retina folded in an extraordinarily marked degree. The surface of the folds which turned towards the cornea was covered by a cellular membrane of varying thickness. According to Kümmell, this membrane could by no means exert a pull on the retina. Considering its form, thickness, and the arrangement and nature of the cells forming it, he concluded that it occurred after the formation of the detachment of the retina. The inflammation was slight. The degeneration process was in front of the equator over the whole uvea, also along the pigment epithelium. From the small cell content of the fluid behind the retina and behind the choroid Kümmell came to the conclusion that it was not an exudate due to inflammation, but a simple transudate. From this we get the following survey of the productive mechanism of a detachment of the retina. The basis is a slow affection of the vascular choroid. By this, on the one hand, the pressure in the vitreous humour region is diminished, on the other hand there is an oversupply of blood in the uveal vessels, which causes transudation. The transudate can force the retina away from its position, while at the same time it is sucked in by the decreased tension of the vitreous humour. The greater the decrease in pressure in the vitreous humour, the greater is the sucking in of the iris-lens diaphragm, which is revealed as an increase in depth of the anterior chamber. The separation from the choroid will be increased if the sclerotic is rigid. The large quantity of protein in the transudate increases its specific gravity and so makes possible its alterations in position. A re-attachment is possible, if the subretinal fluid decreases as a result of a rise in the pressure of the vitreous humour and if strings in the vitreous humour which might prevent this are not present. If the pressure of the vitreous humour rises too quickly, the result is high pressure in the eye, because the fluid has no time to be sucked up quickly. Then, of course, secondary retinal cords hinder a re-attachment to the choroid. The fact that retinal detachment does not occur with every decrease of tension probably depends on the condition of the vitreous and on the delicate attachment of the pigment epithelium to the rods and cones.

It may be concluded that low tension alone is insufficient to produce a detachment, unless the low tension is very marked and occurs suddenly from the loss of solid vitreous, as in Baurmann's case, or unless some degeneration of the choroid or retina exists. It is possible to get hypotony without detachment, and detachment with normal tension. Wessely (1922), as a result of his experiments, concludes that vitreous loss alone is insufficient to cause detachment of the retina. If, however, this loss was accompanied by a choroidal lesion (e.g. a scald), a detachment of the retina followed. Baurmann (1929), when discussing the detachments which follow extraction of the lens, remarks that they are not more likely to occur even if a considerable amount of vitreous is lost. He believes that when detachment does develop in these eyes, it is due to some inflammatory process in the choroid. According to his views the vitreous plays only a passive rôle in the development of retinal detachment. Vail (1920) considers that if there is degeneration of the pars ciliaris retinae as a result of choroiditis, any slight damage due, for example, to dazzling, strain, etc., may arrest the formation of aqueous, lower the tension, and so cause choroidal hyperaemia with an effusion of hypertonic fluid. An attempt to produce a similar state has been made by various operators in an endeavour to lower the tension in absolute glaucoma. It is hoped by them that repeated and extensive cauterisation of the sclera near the limbus will produce atrophy of the ciliary body (Curran, 1924, 1925; Shahan, 1921).

Weekers (1925) agrees that not simply hypotony but a choroidal lesion is the underlying basis of most retinal detachments. He adds that the presence of low tension points to the persistence of the uveal lesion which provoked the detachment of the retina. This brings us to consider the fourth theory.

THE THEORY OF EXUDATION

From its origin this theory has been associated with the name of A. von Graefe. He considered a serous choroiditis to be the primary lesion in the majority of "spontaneous" detachments of the retina. Leber tells us that in the pre-ophthalmoscope days, detachment of the retina, being only recognised after excision, was known as "hydropisie souschoroidienne" (Graefe-Saemisch). This theory brings the mechanism of spontaneous detachment into line with that which explains the formation of fluid in a detachment due to a choroidal sarcoma. Here fluid is secreted under a pressure which exceeds that of the vitreous chamber. Leber considered that this fluid came not only from the vascular tumour itself, but also from the choroidal vessels where the tumour pressed on the veins, and so caused obstruction. This theory applies similarly to the fluid found at times with gliomata of the retina.

A brief consideration of the usual contents of the subretinal or the inter-retinal space may help us to understand this theory. Either a clear or a turbid fluid, or a haemorrhage is present.

INTER-RETINAL FLUID. If this fluid were identical with vitreous, support would be given to the views of Leber and Gonin. But one obvious difference is its greater specific gravity, due to the greater albumen content of inter-retinal fluid. The majority of observers consider that its higher specific gravity is the cause of its descent to the lower pole of the eye. It is also difficult to understand the passage of vitreous upwards through a rent in the upper part of the retina, which is usually the first to be detached. In one eye Kümmel (1921) described how the passage of the inter-retinal fluid into the vitreous through a tear was seen, showing increased pressure in the inter-retinal space. That this occurs is suggested by the fact that the edges of most retinal tears are turned inwards towards the vitreous. Almost certainly in this eye the fluid arose as an effusion. It is further evidence of the fact that not all so-called spontaneous detachments are produced by the same mechanism. Fuchs (1920) states that "subretinal" fluid injected into the eye can produce an inflammation. By such an injection he has caused irritation of the choroid and iris and subsequent iritis. He considers that the foci of inflammation in the uveal tract found in a myopic detachment are due to the subretinal fluid. Probably this occurs only when subretinal fluid arises as an inflammatory exudate from the choroid. One must ask whether vitreous would remain unchanged when lying in a pocket, between the retina and the choroid. If it is not vitreous, as is suggested by Kümmell, is it altered vitreous? If part of the vitreous is degenerate, or if it exudes fluid as a reaction to traumatic or other influences, and a tear is present, it will be this fluid vitreous which passes through and raises up the retina. After some time changes may occur in this fluid and it may bear little resemblance to vitreous itself. The more fluid part may then be absorbed and the remainder form a thick gummy deposit like that found in old experimental detachments. Therefore the dissimilarity of the contents of the two spaces cannot disprove the origin of the subretinal fluid from vitreous. One knows that, as time goes on, the subretinal fluid loses its turbid appearance, and becomes transparent. The passage of a narrow beam of light through the subretinal space in old detachments proves it to be almost optically empty. An image of the source of light is then clearly seen on the pigment epithelium. This can be demonstrated by Gullstrand's binocular ophthalmoscope. Friedenwald (1927, 1929) finds that this effect is most easily obtained with the ophthalmoscope, recently described by him. Masuda (1921), with a special apparatus, has produced in rabbits' eyes retinal oedema, retinal tears, and small detachments of the retina, all due to the experimental formation of inter-retinal fluid.

SUBRETINAL OR INTER-RETINAL HAEMORRHAGE. Many writers have described inter-retinal haemorrhage as a cause of retinal detachment. Such a haemorrhage usually arises as an ordinary retinal haemorrhage which later bursts through into the inter-retinal space (Stanka, 1923; Orlandini, 1922; Gourfein-Welt, 1923). The relative frequency of this after trauma is undoubted. Segi (1923) and Ten Doeschate (1926) report detachment of the retina in purpura haemorrhagica. In the latter's patient, bilateral detachment of the retina occurred, and death followed four days later. Bilateral detachment has been found in children after violent blowing of the nose, and after whooping-cough (Steffan, 1873). Inter-retinal haemorrhage was found to be the cause. The fact that this occurs so rarely suggests some predisposition in these cases as an essential additional factor for the development of detachment. Certain inter-retinal haemorrhages, which affect the macular area, appear to be absorbed in stages. The successive stages are shown by the appearance and disappearance of pigment rings limiting the haemorrhage (Reichling, 1930). Concentric ring-like folds have been described around small macular detachments. These were transient and varied with the degree of re-attachment (Frenkel, 1920; Cassidy and Gifford, 1922).

Weekers considers that the outflow of subretinal fluid plays the main part in the production of detachment of the retina. Gonin disagrees, stating that this theory will explain neither the sudden origin of detachments of the retina nor the habitual superior origin of detachment of the retina.

Before proceeding further it will be wise to consider a theory formulated to explain the presence and the increase in quantity of fluid in the inter-retinal space. It is the diffusion theory.

THE INFLUENCE OF OSMOSIS. The diffusion theory of Rählmann assumes three conditions. Firstly a fluid vitreous is necessary. Normal vitreous has been found to be 98·5 per cent. water. Secondly the retina must act as an animal membrane. Thirdly the fluid in the choroid must possess colloidal properties. It is known that any fluid already in the interretinal space due to a choroidal or retinal lesion has a high albumen and a low saline content. Therefore, in accordance with the laws of diffusion, a flow of the small crystalloid molecules will occur from the more saline fluid in the vitreous into the inter-retinal space. Stallard quotes Scherl's estimation (1893) of the albumen content of effusion in acute choroiditis. This he found was 8·99 per cent., which is about twice as high as the normal albumen content of the fluid in lymphatic vessels. This is in accordance with the teaching of physiology, that there is a greater proteid material content in fluid effused during a state of inflammation than that which forms as a result of pressure in normal physiological circumstances (Halliburton).

There is no evidence to show that osmosis takes place through the living retina. The marked difference in the albumen content on the two sides of the retina in cases of sarcoma suggests that, if it occurs at all, osmosis plays only a small part. A marked difference in osmotic pressure might cause an increase in an already established retinal separation. It would be unlikely to cause a tear in the retina unless it was adherent to the choroid because of previous inflammation.

That the lesion is mainly choroidal is supported by much microscopical work done on eyes with long-standing detachments of the retina. It must also be remembered that the retina is more or less involved in most choroidal inflammations. A fibrinous exudation into the subretinal space will cause adhesions, but a serous effusion may lead to the separation of the two layers.

ASSOCIATION WITH NEPHRITIS. Retinal detachment is relatively common in nephritis, especially if the retina and the choroid are grossly affected, as in the toxaemias of pregnancy. This association is another of the very numerous clinical findings first described by von Graefe (1855). Ochi's (1921) and Hanssen's (1929) recent work on eyes, with detachment of the retina due to renal retinitis, is very striking. Even in these cases the retina, apart from haemorrhage and oedema round the disc, showed little change. The choroid was very degenerate. The chorio-capillaris showed hyaline degeneration and the pigment cells were swollen, or had entirely disappeared. When Verderame (1911) examined histologically an eye, which one year earlier had shown a detachment during pregnancy, he found little retinal change, but the choroidal vessels were very sclerosed.

The various pigment changes seen at times in this condition show the depth of the lesion and the manner in which the choroid may be involved. These have recently been described by Fuchs (1930). Friedenwald considers that a raised intracranial pressure in chronic nephritis can increase the retinal changes by impeding the lymphatic drainage. The choroidal and subretinal effusions will not be affected by this obstruction. They are due directly to the nephritis itself. Foster Moore (1925) collected forty-four detachments of the retina in eyes with renal retinitis. These are due to vascular degeneration and a generalised tendency to oedema. As Fisher has said they are "little more than an expression in the retina and the subretinal space of the oedema which is liable to occur in lax tissues with these general diseases". The most instructive of these are those due to the retinitis of pregnancy. Here there is a sudden onset, a marked effusion, and if the cause is removed, a sudden relief. Detachments are commoner in this form of retinitis than in any true form of renal retinitis. As one would expect there is an effusion, usually bilateral, into the subretinal space, especially in the lower pole. If the patient survives and if pregnancy is terminated, re-attachment is common. In Foster Moore's series 60 per cent. of those associated with pregnancy recovered, while of the remainder only 15 per cent. were reported as having recovered. Of twenty-one patients analysed by Fry (1929) the condition was bilateral in fifteen. Detachment was found in nine primiparas and eleven multiparas. Eighteen patients showed re-attachment, and in four of these this occurred by the end of the fourth day. Hill (1924) reported a patient who recovered from a bilateral detachment, but when the condition recurred at the second pregnancy, only one retina became re-attached. Foster Moore has reported the absorption of inter-retinal fluid in eight days, from the time of its discovery, three days after the removal of twelve pints of ascitic fluid. Foster Moore considers that detachment of the retina does not occur in generalised oedema, apart from retinitis.

ASSOCIATION WITH INFLAMMATION. One is struck with the diverse forms of inflammatory foci, ocular and otherwise, which have been reported as causes of detachment of the retina. In recent years detachments have been reported in association with pansinusitis (Barrenechea, 1922), nasal sepsis (Algan and Coulet, 1925), and orbital cellulitis (Becker, 1922). Becker draws attention to the fact that von Graefe (1854) was the first to report detachment of the retina in orbital cellulitis. One of his own cases was fatal, and the sub-retinal fluid was found to be serous. In another, the detachment of the retina cleared up four weeks after draining an adjacent suppurative focus. Cramer (1922) has described retinal detachment with tenonitis, Somogyi (1925) and Heine (1922) with irido-cyclitis, and Pichler (1925) with episcleritis. Choroidal exudation is considered to be the explanation of the occasional development of detachment of the retina in malaria (Terson, 1903), in typhus (Marin Amat, 1920), in gout by Greeff (1929), and in rheumatism by Schreiber (1920). Greeff's explanation of the part played by urates is worthy of mention. He considers that they are deposited at sites which have poor assimilation, owing to a poor blood supply. For this reason deposits are formed in the sclera. These excite an inflammatory reaction, in which the vascular choroid takes part. An effusion occurs which pushes the retina away. Some writers claim that even detachments occurring in myopia are due to infection. The presence of precipitates on the posterior corneal surface and signs of iritis in myopic detachments convinced Heine (1924, 1928) that tuberculosis or some other infection is the cause. Though Schreiber (1922) considered that most detachments in myopia are due to traction, yet he was able to report two which were probably due to exudation from the choroid. This exudation was "a purely myopic dis-

turbance". They were circumscribed, and bullous in appearance, without any sign of a tear, but with a definite tendency
to re-attachment. Lowenstein (1926) states that many detachments in myopia are due to previous attacks of choroiditis which were probably tuberculous in origin. Schall
(1922, p. 236) described a series of detachments of the retina
which he attributed to tuberculosis. He claimed benefit from
tuberculin therapy. Dor (1910) reported five myopic patients
with detachments, which he considered due to a tuberculous
lesion. He claims that three of these were permanently cured
by injections of tuberculin.

Syphilis appears to play no special part in the production
of detachment of the retina. Giesler (1925) found only four
patients with a positive Wassermann reaction amongst 177
with detachment. One must agree with von Hippel (1913)
that these are very exceptional cases. The presence of obvious
irido-cyclitis enables one to distinguish these cases from so-
called simple "spontaneous" detachment of the retina. When
we remember these diverse associations, we are impelled to
believe that many spontaneous detachments of the retina are
due to uveal disease, which in turn is secondary to some
morbid general phenomenon.

The manner in which a "honeycomb" macula or cystic degeneration can develop in the presence of irido-cyclitis has
been mentioned. Vogt (1921) has observed it associated with
neuro-retinitis, nasal sinus involvement, and thrombosis of
the central retinal vein and with detachment.

SECONDARY RETINITIS. Further evidence of the frequent
association of retinal oedema with sepsis is shown by the star-
like exudates which appear at the macula, not only following
injuries but also in irido-cyclitis and interstitial keratitis. This
appearance is due to the formation of folds in the membrana
limitans interna. They are radial to the macula, where this
membrane is attached. This sensitiveness of the retina to the
presence of sepsis in relatively unrelated tissues is important
in a consideration of the development of retinal detachment.

The occurrence of retinal oedema due to the inflammation
of the anterior ocular tissues has been observed by me in a

little girl over a period of five years. During this time she has had two attacks of bilateral irido-cyclitis of moderate severity. There was an interval of three years between these attacks. When the media had cleared sufficiently, one could see a star at each macula. The exudate was arranged in radiate lines composed of white dots. The lines were finer than those seen in renal retinitis. Similar cases have been described by Leeman (1923), Vogt (1917), Reese (1929), and others. It has been described as a result of sinus infection (Gourfein-Welt, 1921; Bockaert, 1920; Siegrist, 1920), influenza (Sallmann, 1921; Danco, 1921), and other diseases. The possible remoteness of the original infection was demonstrated by a patient described by Brown and Barlow (1929). The neuro-retinitis was secondary to a Vincent's anginal infection of the vagina. The appearance of this condition is similar to that described by Leber as stellate retinitis, by Pascheff (1928) as transitory stellate retinitis, and by Kleiber (1930) as pseudo-nephritic stellate retinitis. The association of detachment with a neuro-retinitis, probably septic in origin, is further evidence of the relationship of sepsis, retinal oedema, and detachment (Rea, 1923). The central scotoma found in 37 per cent. of patients with iritis by Lippmann (1921) was probably due to the influence of toxins on the retina. Often owing to the opacities in the media, this is the only means of demonstrating retinal involvement. Microscopic sections of eyes with secondary retinitis have shown the perivascular lymph spaces invaded by lymphocytes. It appears, therefore, that the retina is very sensitive to inflammation of the anterior ocular tissues.

Leber objected to the exudation theory, because of the absence of a rise in tension, as already referred to, and because of the rare finding of any of the usual accompaniments of choroiditis. That effusion from the uveal tract can occur with a minimum of obvious inflammation is shown by a certain type of iritis. It is characterised by a sudden loss of vision, due to the filling of the pupil with exudate, and by an absence of the usual ciliary injection and pain. This form of iritis is one which I have seen only twice. In each patient both eyes were affected, and in neither could any causative septic focus be found. The complaint was sudden loss of vision without pain. On examination, little or no injection was detected. The iris moved slowly and within its pupillary margin there appeared a disc of semi-solid exudate lying on the lens capsule. The iris moved up to its margin and away from it freely, and did not appear congested. The disc disappeared in two or three days, and in neither case has returned. If this can occur with what one considers to be a mild and quiet iritis, a similar sudden lesion may affect any other part of the uveal tract. An effusion from tissues as vascular as are the choroid and the iris can occur suddenly and without obvious signs of inflammation. Therefore not much importance need be attached to the objection made by Leber to the theory of exudation, that evidence of the presence of choroiditis is usually wanting. One is only too apt to consider that an effusion must be extensive to cause a detachment. It is probable that the initial exudate is often not large at all. As has been shown, a very mild lesion can produce exudation. One would not expect to see the focus itself, for the detachment hides it. The other changes, viz. leucocytosis of the aqueous, fine wrinkling of Descemet's membrane and bedewing of the corneal endothelium were practically unknown until the slit-lamp revealed them. The lowered tension, so common in detachment of the retina, may be directly due to the uveitis.

It is interesting here to recall the phenomenon described by Weekers (1924) under the title of "consensual ophthalmotonic reaction". By experiments he was able to observe a reflex dilatation of uveal vessels in one eye as a result of the vascular congestion which he produced in the other eye. If the latter was intense, exudation from the choroid was found in both eyes (Leplat, 1924).

DETACHMENT OF THE RETINA IN SYMPATHETIC OPHTHALMITIS. Leber described several examples of this association. The actual cause of the detachment is almost certainly a choroidal exudate. Haab, Groenouw and Peters, in describing this appearance, referred to it as a "phantom tumour". Pascheff (1928) has recently described a patient with detachment of the retina, due to sympathetic ophthalmitis, which was completely cured. Aykai (1921) described a similar detachment which became re-attached after the exciting eye was excised. Salzmann (1921) described an eye in which the detachment spread forwards and involved the orbiculus ciliaris as well. Weisner (1927) described a detachment of the choroid with normal tension at the beginning of sympathetic ophthalmitis.

INFLUENCE OF LIGHT AND HEAT. It is not uncommon after an eclipse of the sun for inadequately protected observers to develop retinal oedema, a macular hole, and even a detachment (Harman and Macdonald, 1922).

Exposure to intense light produced a macular detachment in Rauh's patient (1927). Jess (1920) showed that the retinal epithelium was mainly affected in exposure during a solar eclipse. Such findings are of special interest in the light of Czerny's experiments (*Ann. d'Ocul.* xxxv, p. 252). He produced disintegration of the retinal pigment epithelium and a detachment by concentrating solar rays on the retinae of certain animals. He considered this a possible cause of macular detachment clinically. It is probable that Plateau, the physicist of Ghent, became blind from macular degeneration. This followed gazing at the mid-day sun when carrying out experiments on vision (Bayliss). The lesion produced by such exposure is almost purely thermal in origin. The pigment epithelium shares with the skin the capacity to absorb light rays and degrade them into heat. Twenty-six years ago Birch-Hirschfeld (1904) reported retinal changes due to ultra-violet rays. All other observers failed to find these until recently W. S. and P. M. Duke-Elder (1929) conclusively proved their existence. They showed that these short-waved rays acted mainly on the ganglion cells, and that their influence diminished progressively inwards towards the choroid. In thermal lesions the rods and cones are most affected, and the changes progressively decrease in intensity outwards. Probably both thermal and short-wave rays are effective, when retinal damage is due to electrical or to lightning flashes (Roy, 1929).

EXPERIMENTAL WORK. Further support is given to this theory by the experimental work of Wessely (1922) and Weekers (1924). The former using hot steam and the latter a cautery produced detachments due to choroidal exudation. These detachments followed the course of detachments observed clinically. The upper or primary detachment tended to heal, leaving atrophy and pigmentation to mark its site, whilst the lower or secondary detachment persisted and the fluid tended to recur after evacuation (Wessely). The fluid was found to be highly albuminous, viscous, more or less cloudy and either grey, green or yellowish. Sometimes it was found to contain cholesterin crystals and flakes of fibrin. I have repeated their experiments on a series of twenty-four rabbits. My findings agree with theirs, in all points, except the tendency for the secondary detachment to clear up. The fluid appeared to me to be absorbed slowly, and not to persist for as long a time as Weekers stated. If one cauterises the eye of a rabbit, one can with the ophthalmoscope detect immediately an area of retinal oedema. In a few minutes a globular detachment appears which migrates in part to the lower pole about the fourth day. Subretinal fluid does not persist above or laterally, but it can be withdrawn in a degenerate state from the lower pole two or three months later; whereas, when one cauterises the inferior pole, the globular detachment which forms clears up more rapidly. It appears as if the cauterisation which produces the detachment also produces the conditions which make its rapid absorption possible. It appears also as if a similar vascular reaction would explain the good results which followed the old operation of cauterisation.

As long as the congestion is acute, it need only be slight or localised to cause a detachment of the retina. Weekers's microscopical sections show slight scleral and episcleral disturbance, but considerable vascular congestion in the choroid. The retina at first sight is only slightly affected, but fluid is seen between the pigment layer and the rods and cones. In very marked cases of choroidal congestion even the pigment layer is stripped from the lamina vitrea.

Because of the shallowness of the detachment of the retina above, due to the normal fixation of the retina to the choroid at the ora serrata, re-attachment can easily occur when the bulk of the exudate descends. In some eyes the choroid was found detached from the sclera on one side and from the pigment epithelium on the other. Weekers aptly compares the marked choroidal lesion which may be small with the extensive lid oedema and chemosis sometimes seen in folliculitis. "These facts", he says, "are explained by the anatomy of the part"—an area existing of lowered resistance to the forces which make for cleavage. As has been seen, Leber, Nordenson and Gonin insisted on the constancy of anterior choroiditis in eyes with detachment of the retina. Their interpretation however was different. According to them, the choroiditis caused first a vitreous degeneration in its vicinity. The retraction of the vitreous then pulled on and tore the retina, and so allowed the vitreous to escape under it.

In my experiments vitreous bands occurred only if the three coats of the eye were cauterised, allowing vitreous to escape at the time. In certain of these, fine strands developed, which probably later would have produced detachment of the retina. With the ophthalmoscope one could observe the round hole in the retina made with the cautery, and its presence appeared to have no retarding effect on the adhering of the retina to the choroid.

The tendency for the upper or primary detachment to re-attach explains, according to Weekers, the rarity of detachment of the retina in myopic eyes with signs of old diffuse choroiditis. The retina is fixed more firmly than before at the site of the scars. One attack of choroiditis constitutes a risk of detachment of the retina. Once healed, it becomes a protection against it. Five weeks after cauterisation, a section of the eye will show that the choroid and the retina are adherent, both being atrophic. It will also be observed that pigment has spread into the choroid and sclera.

Whilst Gonin holds that tears are causative and that their persistence attributes to indefinite continuation of detachment of the retina, Weekers considers that they are merely accidents in the course of the development of a detachment. He has observed them in only some of his clinical and experimental detachments. At times he has found tears in the lower retina detached by the descent of the exudate. He considers that tears occur when choroiditis is particularly acute and consequently retinal damage is great.

As the exudate slides down it separates the two retinal layers, causing so little upset that, apart from occasional folds, there is nothing to be seen with the ophthalmoscope. Weekers was struck by the slight alteration in the vitreous. Occasionally, if cauterisation was excessive, choroidal exudate passed through the retina and produced a limited vitreous detachment.

The part played by the uvea is shown by a study of the tension in Weekers's experiments. There was always a preliminary rise followed by prolonged hypotony. He has observed clinically an initial but transient rise in tension in detachment of the retina. This is a point not usually recognised. Its importance is emphasised when one recalls Leber's objections to the exudation theory. He objected to it mainly on two grounds. Firstly, if a sudden exudate is the cause of the detachment, the tension should be raised immediately. This rise should continue until the increase of ocular contents is counterbalanced by the loss of fluid from the eye. Secondly, as a rule, there is no sign of ocular inflammation in the suddenly arising detachments. If choroiditis with effusion is the cause, he expects manifestations of uveitis. The finding of Weekers is very important in the light of Leber's first objection.

If one injects some sodium fluorescein under the skin of a rabbit, one eye of which has been cauterised, the cauterised eye becomes more strongly and more rapidly coloured, because the uveal vessels are more dilated and more permeable. As the tension falls the time taken for colour to appear grows less until the tension has returned to normal, when both eyes colour together. The detachment of the retina persists, however, at a maximum. Therefore the changes in tension must be independent of it, and tension must rise with the initial enormous choroidal congestion and consequent exudation, and fall later as a result of excessive aqueous elimination. During this period of low tension histologically the choroidal vessels appear dilated and the fluorescein test reveals a state of marked vascular permeability. The colour appears quickly, as a cloud, in the lower part of the anterior chamber. It disappears quickly also because of the extra activity of the "émonctoires" of the aqueous. After fourteen days tension it is normal again, and the uveal congestion has gone. This period represents the time necessary for the restoration of normal uveal circulation by the cicatrisation and healing of the superficial burn. There are therefore three stages: the first of raised tension, and the rapid and marked appearance of fluorescein; the second of low tension, during which fluorescein appears very slowly; and the third of normal tension, when fluorescein will appear equally and at the same time in each eye. The independence of the detachment of the retina and the variations in tension are shown by the fact that during these three stages the detachment of the retina usually remains maximal. The variations in tension depend above all on the vascular variations in the uvea and the effect of this on the flow of aqueous, *i.e.* the cause of the detachment is also the cause of the variations in tension, though these are mutually independent. In the third stage, the vascular variations having ceased, the tension remains stable, but the detachment persists. Therefore, clinically, hypotony shows persistence of the uveal lesions which produced the detachment. It is therefore a bad omen.

It is of interest to compare with these findings the effects which Amsler (1929) noticed when he performed Gonin's operation of ignipuncture on a blind glaucomatous eye. There was a marked rise in tension from 40 to 60 mm. during the first day. This was followed by a marked and prolonged hypotony (16 mm.).

It is well at this stage to refer to Magitot's ingenious theory to explain variations of tension. He considers that the ganglion cells of Müller in the choroid form a nerve centre which regulates the size of the vessels. The tension is maintained by the equilibrium established between two factors, viz. the relative size of the "supplying" arteries and that of the "draining" veins. In normal conditions this equilibrium will be assured by the integrity of the nerve centre. Any derangement of this such as massage, cauterisation, paracentesis of the anterior chamber, etc., will upset the normal balance. He explains the varying effects on the ocular tension that trauma may produce in a similar way. If there is inhibition of the nerve cells there will be passive dilatation of the choroidal vessels with rise in tension. Excitation of these cells will produce a fall in tension by constriction of the same vessels.

By such means one can explain the vascular turgescence observed anatomically after cauterisation and the short but considerable rise in tension.

SUMMARY OF PATHOGENESIS

In the past too many attempts have been made to include all retinal detachments without an obvious cause under one heading, and to attribute to them one productive mechanism. We are nearer to the truth if we consider a variation in the actual causes. No one condition *sine qua non* is to be found. For, though a hole can be found in the majority of detached retinae, yet detachments do occur without hole formation, and at times holes are seen without detachments. Though the ocular tension is usually reduced, yet it may be normal or at times increased. Though hypotony, especially if due to the loss of normal vitreous, may lead to a detachment, yet hypotony alone need not necessarily produce a detachment, as is proved by a study of diabetic coma. Though choroidal effusion can so easily produce retinal separation under experimental conditions, yet this will not account for all detachments met with in clinical practice.

The finding of a hole in almost every detachment, as stated by Gonin and Vogt, gives such an appearance greater importance in pathogenesis than it had before. Vogt has stated, "The results of operation produce the proof that the retinal hole is the cause of spontaneous detachment". The good results following the closing of such holes by ignipuncture are beyond doubt. But, though it appears probable that hole formation may be the exciting event in the history of vitreous and retinal degeneration which leads to detachment, and its closure the means of cure, yet the benefit of the neighbouring firm adhesions, that form between vitreous, retina and choroid as a result of the operation, must not be overlooked. These adhesions, and the occasional incidental closing of a hole, probably explain the successes from the older operation of cautery puncture. Neither must it be forgotten that the response of the tissues to the cauterisation increases their absorptive capacity. The vascular reaction which follows the operation resembles the state which exists when an inflammatory focus produces a detachment by the exudation of fluid. This reaction is probably one explanation why the prognosis is better in such cases than in those due to a different mechanism. The experimental detachments in animals, already referred to, revealed not only an innate tendency towards spontaneous re-attachment, but also a decided capacity for retinal tears to heal.

It can therefore be concluded that, though the results of ignipuncture are beyond doubt, one is not qualified yet in assuming that in all cases the tear was instrumental in producing the detachment now cured by the operation which has closed the tear.

Vogt wisely distinguishes rents from holes. The latter he considers are due to the tearing away of a disc-like area of retina by an adherent and degenerate vitreous framework. These holes are round or oval. At times when the disc of retina remains attached at one point, it appears as if the hole had a lid (*ein Deckel*) and is horseshoe-shaped. In one patient Vogt detected a movement of the lid when the eye was rotated (1930 *a*). At other times he has found the lid at some distance from the hole (1930 *b*). He has frequently observed these holes in fundi which showed no cystoid degeneration, and therefore he considered the vitreous framework the agent, just as it certainly is in a detachment due to the discission of secondary cataract. Further support for this theory is given by the fact that the lid is always turned away from the choroid and towards the vitreous. The edges of the hole, too, appear drawn inwards (1930 *c*). The lid which always appears smaller than the hole, as a result of contraction, is often an aid in finding the hole. Vogt considers that the tear is actually produced by shaking movements of the vitreous during ocular rotation or bodily efforts, rather than by a long-continued traction. The occurrence of detachments after movements, and the occasional re-attachments which occur after prolonged rest, support this conception. He considers that spontaneous cures are due to the innate tendency of these holes, as of wounds elsewhere, to heal.

At other times Vogt admits holes are due to cystoid degeneration. He has found that a series of holes may be limited to one quadrant, or to one-half of a retina, while the remainder appears healthy. Gonin considers that detachments are due either to this cause or to a traumatic rent. He, however, emphasises the importance of the part played by a previous focal attack of retino-choroiditis in the equatorial region in producing adhesions between the retina and the vitreous.

In detachment due to cystoid degeneration there is no need to postulate inflammatory changes as Leber did. The preponderance of people over fifty years of age and of myopes, amongst the patients with retinal detachment, is largely due to the presence of cystoid degeneration. Vogt describes three old non-myopic patients, in whom he considered detachment was due to the degeneration of senility alone. In these he made the diagnosis of senile "amotio". Often there is a history of some slight almost unnoticed trauma, or physical strain. Possibly in a myopic eye, predisposed by degeneration and hypotony, some trivial cause is all that is necessary to excite a detachment. It has been seen that traumatic detachments may be either active or passive. When a cicatricial band by drawing the retina away tears it and the escape of vitreous is permitted, the retinal separation is active. If, however, the passage of the fluid through a hole is primary, and the retinal elevation results from this, the detachment is considered to be passive. It is interesting to recall, however, that only 16 per cent. of patients in Stallard's series gave a history of trauma. This and Cords's comment, that it is only very rarely that one sees a detachment due to contusion, suggest that in the past we have been too much occupied with trauma as a cause.

Vogt considers that as a rule a contusion produces a tear near the ora serrata in the thinnest part of the retina and that, when vitreous filters through, the retina becomes detached. He has seen, after trauma, vesicle-like detachments on the summit of which tears were found. During the subsequent days or weeks, he has watched these detachments as they became complete. He was struck by the similarity of the appearances found frequently in non-traumatic detachments. When early they were vesicle-like with a tear on the summit. The exudate gradually sank away from the torn area, and produced a total detachment. The degeneration of the retina is shown, Vogt believes, by the tendency of the hole to increase in size, and by its shredded margin. "To contest the causal connection between a spontaneous detachment and this hole formation is denying the simplest fact." Vogt accounts for the fact that retinal tears, which lead to detachment, are usually situated in the upper pole by the greater specific gravity of the retina. If it is assumed that all quadrants of the retina are equally capable of tearing, then, because of man's erect posture, degenerate parts in the upper pole of the relatively heavy retina will "feel a pull" first.

The excellent results reported by Gonin and Vogt from the operation of "ignipuncture", or obliterating cauterisation of the retinal aperture, are proof of the part played by such a hole in the mechanism which produces a detachment. The actual cause of any one hole may vary. It may be due to retinal degeneration, the traction of a degenerate and adherent vitreous, or directly to trauma. It may at times also be due to the lytic effect of the subretinal fluid in those detachments which are due to the formation of an exudate, or it may be due to a sudden exudate, if the retina and choroid are adherent from the previous inflammation. Certainly the latter type exists, and the theories of Hanssen, Vogt and Gonin cannot explain it. Neither do the authors of these theories deny the occurrence of detachment by exudation. Vogt does not say that all detachments are due to degeneration of the vitreous framework and a retinal tear, and nothing else. Though one gains from those who write about these theories the impression that each author considers his theory capable of universal application, this is incorrect and misleading. Vogt considers that hole formation is rare in detachments due to choroidal inflammation, and that the recognition of such detachments is simplified if one finds other signs of inflammation.

It appears therefore that, in the absence of adequate trauma, the retina may be pushed from the choroid by a tumour, haemorrhage, or exudate, or may be lifted from it as fluid passes underneath it through a retinal hole. This hole may be due either to cystoid degeneration or to the traction of an adherent and degenerate vitreous. The presence of definite vitreous bands is rare, and is only a very infrequent cause of retinal detachment. The rarity of tears and the positive findings of transillumination, of tonometry, and of microscopy, enable us as a rule to exclude a haemorrhage or a tumour. The absence of any sign of cystoid degeneration, or the finding of a rounded hole, especially if accompanied by a lid, will make possible a recognition of a detachment due to the mechanism described by Vogt.

It further appears that amongst cases of "idiopathic" or spontaneous detachments of the retina there are two main groups. One is essentially due to degeneration, whether it be in the form of cystoid changes in the retina, vitreous liquefaction, or alterations in both these tissues after equatorial retino-choroiditis. The other group is due to choroidal effusion, and the appearance of a retinal tear is incidental rather than essential as it is in the former group. The subretinal fluid is albuminous and less watery than that found in examples of the degenerative group in which the subretinal fluid closely resembles fluid vitreous. Detachments due to choroidal effusion have a better prognosis than those due to retinal and vitreous degeneration. The lesion that produces the detachment produces a reaction which tends to cure the detachment, and even to close a retinal tear. Such a type is very similar to the experimental detachments produced by a burn or scald. Between these two main groups there is an intermediate group, where both degeneration and effusion combine as agents of causation.

It is hoped that Vogt's statement (1929), that spontaneous detachments are the most common, will soon be out of date. For spontaneous conditions are simply those the productive mechanisms of which are unrecognised. We have no more right for considering them to be spontaneous, than Cinderella's prince would have had for so explaining the arrival of her shoe. It is only by hard work that the mysteries of that fairy god-mother, Nature, will be revealed, and her ways of strewing stray shoes solved.

REFERENCES

THE THEORY OF DISTENSION AND THE ASSOCIATION OF MYOPIA

1857. v. GRAEFE, A. *Arch. f. Ophthal.* **2**, 277.
1897. OTTO, F. *Ibid.* **43**, 2, 323.
1899. v. HIPPEL, E. *Ibid.* **49**, 2, 387.
1904–8 *a*. PARSONS, J. H. *The Pathology of the Eye*, **3**, part 1, 920.
1904–8 *b*. —— *Ibid.* 917.
1915. HELMING. Inaug. Diss. Giessen.
1916. SEIBLE. *Klin. Monatsbl. f. Augenheilk.* **56**, 587.
1919. GONIN, J. *Ann. d'Ocul.* **156**, 281.
1920. HELMING. *Ophthal. Year Book* (abstract), **16**, 192
1920. SCHREIBER, L. *Arch. f. Ophthal.* **103**, 750.
1920. GILBERT, W. *Arch. f. Augenheilk.* **86**, 282.
1920. FUCHS. *Arch. de Oftal. Hisp. Amer.* **20**, 293.
1921. DOR, L. *Rev. gén. d'ophtal.* Oct. **35**, 441.
1922. UHTHOFF, W. *Deutsch. med. Wochenschr.* **28**, 115.
1923. KREKELER, F. *Arch. f. Augenheilk.* Sept. **93**, 144.
1923. LAUBER, H. *Klin. Monatsbl. f. Augenheilk.* **70**, 246.
1925. HANSSEN, R. *Ibid.* **74**, 778.
1925. —— *Ibid.* **75**, 344.
1928. COMBERG, W. *Ber. ü. d. Versamml. d. deutsch. ophthal. Gesellsch.* **74**, 126.
1928–9. LEVINSOHN, G. *Ibid.* **74**, 131; *Arch. f. Augenheilk.* 1929, **102**, 308.
1928. LEVINSOHN, F. *Klin. Monatsbl. f. Augenheilk.* **80**, 56.
1928. CLAUSEN, W. *Ibid.* **80**, 510.
1928. REHSTEINER, K. *Arch. f. Ophthal.* **120**, 282.
1929. NEWMAN, F. *Amer. Jl. of Ophthal.* Sept. **12**, 714.

CYSTOID DEGENERATION OF THE RETINA

1855. BLESSIG, R. *De Retinae Structura*, Dorpat, 47.
1857. MÜLLER, H. *Zeit. f. Wissensch. Zool.* **8**, 1.
1865. IWANOFF, A. *Arch. f. Ophthal.* part 1, **11**, 135.
1876. NETTLESHIP, E. *Ophthal. Hosp. Rep. London*, **7**, 3.
1900. GREEFF, R. *Arch. f. Augenheilk.* **40**, 99; *Graefe-Saemisch Handbuch*, 2nd edn., part 1, **1**, 5.
1912. SALZMANN, M. *Anatomy and Physiology of the Human Eye*, 84.
1919. GONIN, J. *Klin. Monatsbl. f. Augenheilk.* **63**, 295.
1921. —— *Vienna Ophthal. Congress*, August, 273.
1921. FUCHS, A. *Arch. f. Ophthal.* **105**, 333.
1923. —— *Ophthal. Year Book*, **19**, 223.
1924. v. BERGER, F. *Klin. Monatsbl. f. Augenheilk.* **72**, 837.
1925. HANSSEN, R. *Ibid.* **74**, 778.

1925. HANSSEN, R. *Klin. Monatsbl. f. Augenheilk.* **75**, 344.
1927. OCHI, S. *Amer. Jl. of Ophthal.* **10**, 161.
1928. GONIN, J. *Zeitschr. f. Augenheilk.* **63**, 370.
1928. —— *Klin. Monatsbl. f. Augenheilk.* (abstract), **80**, 127.
1929. PRESSBURGER, E. *Zeitschr. f. Augenheilk.* **68**, 331.
1929. KAPUCZINSKI. *Trans. 13th Internat. Ophthal. Congress, Amsterdam.*

ASSOCIATION OF TRAUMA

1891. SCHEFFELS, O. *Arch. f. Augenheilk.* **22**, 308.
1915. STÄHLI, J. *Klin. Monatsbl. f. Augenheilk.* Sept.
1918. FRANCISCO, F. *Cronica Med. Quirurgica de la Habana* (Dec.).
1919. AMMANN, E. *Klin. Monatsbl. f. Augenheilk.* **63**, July.
1919. BREUCKNER, A. *Zeitschr. f. Augenheilk.* **41**, 255.
1919. LACROIX, A. *Arch. d'Ophtal.* **33**, 439.
1919. ROCHAT, G. F. *Ophthal. Year Book*, **15**, 160.
1919. VOGT, A. *Klin. Monatsbl. f. Augenheilk.* **62**, 619.
1920. FUCHS, E. *Ibid.* **64**, 1.
1920. McDAVITT, T. *Southern Med. Journal*, **13**, 378.
1921. DUBOIS, H. F. and CUPERUS. *Amer. Jl. of Ophthal.* **4**, 771.
1921. VOGT, A. and KNUESEL, O. *Klin. Monatsbl. f. Augenheilk.* **67**, 513.
1922. BRINTON, A. G. *Amer. Jl. of Ophthal.* **5**, 806.
1922. GIFFORD, S. R. and LA RUE. *Amer. Jl. of Ophthal.* **5**.
1924. NEBLETT, H. C. *Amer. Jl. of Ophthal.* **7**, 564.
1925. REESE, W. S. *Amer. Jl. of Ophthal.* **8**, 371.
1929. CHOU, C. H. *Nat. Med. Jl. China.* **15**, 592.
1929. MARTIN, W. O. *Amer. Jl. of Ophthal.* **12**, 652.
1929. VOGT, A. *Schweiz. med. Wochenschr.* March 23rd, 331.
1930. CORDS, R. *Klin. Monatsbl. f. Augenheilk.* **84**, 222.

THE MECHANISM OF TRAUMA

1854. V. GRAEFE, A. *Arch. f. Ophthal.* **33**, 3, 21.
1869. COWELL, G. *Ophthal. Hosp. Rep. London*, **6**, 4, 255.
1887. HUGHES, H. *Arch. f. Ophthal.* **33**, 3, 21.
1912. GONIN, J. *Ann. d'Ocul.* **147**, 18.
1924. LISTER, Sir W. *Brit. Jl. of Ophthal.* **8**, 1 and 305.
1929. DUBOIS, H. *Ann. d'Ocul.* **166**, 81.

RETINAL TEARS

1869. KNAPP, J. H. *Arch. f. Augenheilk. u. Ohrenheilk.* **1**, 1, 22.
1870. DE WECKER, L. *Traité des malad. du fond de l'œil*, Paris, 153.
1871. NOYES, H. D. *Trans. Amer. Ophthal. Soc.* **8**, 128.
1875. PÄGENSTECHER, H. *Atlas der pathol. Anat. des Augapfels*, Wiesbaden, **28**, 6.
1877. FUCHS, E. *Zehender Monatsbl.* **15**, 422.

1883. SCHWEIGGER, C. *Arch. f. Augenheilk.* **12**, 332.
1887. NORDENSON, E. *Retinal Detachment*, **4**, Wiesbaden.
1890. SCHEFFELS, O. *Arch. f. Augenheilk.* **22**, 308.
1891. HORTSMANN, C. *Ber. über die 21. Vers. der ophthal. Gesell.* 140.
1896. DUNN. *Arch. of Ophthal.* **25**, 1.
1896. NUEL. *Arch. d'Ophtal.* **16**, 164.
1896. COLLINS, E. TREACHER. *Trans. Ophthal. Soc. U.K.* **16**, 81.
1898. ELLERHORST. *Zentralbl. f. pr. Augenheilk.* **22**, 266.
1898. DIMMER, F. *12th Internat. Congress. Ophthal. Moscow*, **11**, 144.
1898. HORTSMANN, C. *Ber. über die 21. Vers. der ophthal. Gesell.* 140.
1900. COLLINS, E. TREACHER. *Trans. Ophthal. Soc. U.K.* **20**, 196.
1900. HAAB, O. *Zeitschr. f. Augenheilk.* **3**, 113.
1900. KUHNT, H. *Ibid.* **3**, 106.
1900. OGILVIE, F. M. *Trans. Ophthal. Soc. U.K.* **20**, 202.
1901. HARMAN, BISHOP. *Ibid.* **21**.
1901. FUCHS, E. *Zeitschr. f. Augenheilk.* **6**, 181.
1902. DOYNE, R. W. *Ophthal. Rev.* 108.
1902. CHEVALLEREAU. *Bull. Soc. d'Ophtal. de Paris.*
1904. DE SCHWEINITZ, G. *Trans. Amer. Ophthal. Soc.* **10**, 228.
1904. HOLDEN, W. A. *Ann. d'Ocul.* (abstract), **132**, 125.
1904. GONIN, J. *Ibid.* **132**, 30.
1906. REIS. *Zeitschr. f. Augenheilk.* **20**, 311.
1906. KÜSEL. *Klin. Monatsbl. f. Augenheilk.* **46**, 2, 464.
1906. DUFOUR and GONIN, J. *Encycl. franç. d'Ophtal.* **6**, 938.
1906. QUINT. *Klin. Monatsbl. f. Augenheilk.* **44**, 134.
1906. GONIN, J. *See* Dufour and Gonin.
1907. COATS, G. *Ophthal. Hosp. Rep.* London, **17**, 69.
1907. TWIETMAYER. *Zeitschr. f. Augenheilk.* **18**, 447.
1908. STOCK. *Klin. Monatsbl. f. Augenheilk.* **46**, 1, 236.
1908. HAAB, O. *Atlas und Grundriss der Ophthal.* **5**.
1908. v. HIPPEL, E. *Arch. f. Ophthal.* **58**, 38.
1908. NOLL. *Arch. f. Augenheilk.* **60**, 254.
1908. KIPP and ALT. *Amer. Jl. of Ophthal.* 225.
1909. ZENTMAYER, W. *Ophthal. Rec.* 198.
1909. PURTSCHER, A. *Zeitschr. f. Augenheilk.* **22**, 215.
1910. MOORE, R. FOSTER. *Trans. Ophthal. Soc. U.K.* **30**, 155.
1911. FUCHS, E. *Arch. f. Ophthal.* **79**, 1, 42.
1912. ZEEMAN, W. P. *Ibid.* **88**, 370.
1914. ELSCHNIG, A. *Arch. f. Augenheilk.* **77**, 6 and 252.
1916. LEBER, TH. *Graefe-Saemisch Handb.* 2nd edn., **7**, part 2, chap. 10, 1396.
1916. STÄHLI, J. *Ophthal. Year Book* (abstract), **12**, 205.
1916. PURTSCHER, A. *Klin. Monatsbl. f. Augenheilk.* **56**, 244.
1918. MAXEY, E. *Amer. Jl. of Ophthal.* **1**, 81.
1919. MIDDLETON, A. B. *Ibid.* **2**, 779.
1919. MAXEY, E. *Amer. Jl. of Ophthal.* **2**, 792.

1919. MASUDA. *Nippon Gank. Zasshi.* July.
1919. v. SZILY. *Deutsch. med. Wochenschr.* **43**, 1214.
1919. SALZMANN, M. *Wiener. med. Wochenschr.* **16**.
1920. HEHR. *Klin Monatsbl. f. Augenheilk.* **64**, 142.
1920. FINNOFF, W. C. *Amer. Jl. of Ophthal.* **3**, 130.
1920. VOGT, A. *Klin. Monatsbl. f. Augenheilk.* **65**, 103.
1921. —— *Ibid.* **66**, 321, 718, 838.
1921–2. WILLIAMSON, F. A. *Amer. Jl. of Ophthal.* **4**, 467; **5**, 139.
1924. VOGT, A. *Klin. Monatsbl. f. Augenheilk.* **72**, 335.
1924. LISTER, Sir W. *Brit. Jl. of Ophthal.* **8**, 1, 2.
1925. VOGT, A. *Münch. med. Wochenschr.* **72**, 1101.
1925. ARCHANGELSKY, W. *Klin. Monatsbl. f. Augenheilk.* **74**, 266.
1926. DEUTSCHMANN, F. *Arch. f. Ophthal.* **117**, 146.
1926. FLEISCHER, J. *Zeitschr. f. Augenheilk.* **68**, 375.
1928. BIRCH-HIRSCHFELD. *Klin. Monatsbl. f. Augenheilk.* **80**, 531.
1928. GONIN, J. *Bull. Soc. d'Ophtal. de Paris*, 275.
1929. ARNOLD, MAX. *Arch. f. Ophthal.* **122**, 299.
1929. SCHIECK, F. *Arch. f. Augenheilk.* **100–1**, 857.
1929 VOGT, A *Schweiz. med. Wochenschr.* 331.
1929. —— *Klin. Monatsbl. f. Augenheilk.* **82**, 619.
1930. —— *Ibid.* **84**, 305.

THEORY OF ATTRACTION

1858. MÜLLER, H. *Anatom. Beiträge z. Ophthal.* **41**, 363.
1876. v. ARLT, F. *Über die Ursachen und die Entstehung der Kurzsichtig-keit*, Wien, 8.
1882. LEBER, TH. *Trans. Internat. Med. Congr.* 7th Session, London, **3**, 15.
1887. NORDENSON, E. *Retinal Detachment*, Wiesbaden, **4**.
1893. RÄHLMANN, E. *Arch. f. Augenheilk.* **27**, 1.
1900. v. HIPPEL, E. *Arch. f. Ophthal.* **51**, 132.
1908. —— *Ibid.* **68**, 38.
1904. GONIN, J. *Ann. d'Ocul.* **132**, 30.
1916. LEBER, TH. *Graefe-Saemisch Handb.* 2nd edn., **7**, part 2, chap. 10.
1920. GONIN, J. *Amer. Jl. of Ophthal.* **3**, 57.
1923. FUCHS, E. *Text-book of Ophthal.* Trans. by Duane, 7th edn., 674.
1923. GONIN, J. *Klin. Monatsbl. f. Augenheilk.* **71**, 232.
1924. HEINE, L. *Ibid.* **72**, 305.
1924. LAUBER, H. *Ibid.* **72**, 547.
1924. ROLLET, E. and ROSNOBLET. *Arch. d'Ophtal.* **41**, 48.
1929. GONIN, J. *Klin. Monatsbl. f. Augenheilk.* **83**, 667.

VITREOUS DETACHMENT

1869. IWANOFF, A. *Arch. f. Ophthal.* **15**, 1.
1914. ERGGELET, M. *Klin. Monatsbl. f. Augenheilk.* **53**, 449.
1916. SINCLAIR, W. W. *Trans. Ophthal. Soc. U.K.* **36**, 373.

1919. PURTSCHER, A. *Zeitschr. f. Augenheilk.* **42**, 256.
1919. ROBERTS, B. H. *Trans. Ophthal. Soc. U.K.* **39**, 371.
1922. LISTER, W. *Amer. Jl. of Ophthal.* **5**, 488.
1922. PILLAT, A. *Klin. Monatsbl. f. Augenheilk.* **69**, 429.
1922. RALSTON, W. and GOAR, E. L. *Amer. Jl. of Ophthal.* **5**, 372.
1923. FUCHS, E. *Text-book of Ophthal.* Trans. by Duane, 7th edn., 654.
1923. GOLDSTEIN, I. *Arch. of Ophthal.* **52**, 271.
1923. GIMBLETT, C. *Proc. Roy. Soc. Med. London*, Jan. 20.
1923. KRAUPA, E. *Klin. Monatsbl. f. Augenheilk.* **70**, 716.
1923. REA, L. *Proc. Roy. Soc. Med. London*, Jan. 20.
1923. RINGLE, C. A. *Amer. Jl. of Ophthal.* **6**, 603.
1924. COMBERG, W. *Klin. Monatsbl. f. Augenheilk.* **72**, 692.
1924. KRAUPA, E. *Ibid.* **72**, 476.
1924. SANTA-CRUZ, B. *Arch. de Oftal. Hisp. Amer.* **24**, 575, 593.
1925. KRAUPA, E. *Klin. Monatsbl. f. Augenheilk.* **75**, 708.
1925. MEISNER, M. *Ibid.* **74**, 778.
1925. PILLAT, A. *Zeitschr. f. Augenheilk.* **57**, 347.
1926. ISAKOWITZ, J. *Klin. Monatsbl. f. Augenheilk.* **77**, 121.

CRITICISM OF TRACTION THEORY

1915. HANSSEN, R. *Klin. Monatsbl. f. Augenheilk.* **56**, 545.
1919. —— *Ibid.* **63**, 295.
1920. FUCHS, E. *Arch. de Oftal. Hisp. Amer.* **20**, 293.
1921. —— *Arch. f. Ophthal.* **104**, 230.
1923. VOGT, A. *Zeitschr. f. Augenheilk.* **49**, 67.
1924. COMBERG, W. *Klin. Monatsbl. f. Augenheilk.* **72**, 692.
1924. VOGT, A. *Ibid.* **72**, 212.
1925. KOBY, F. E. *Ibid.* **74**, 196.
1925. WEEKERS, L. *Arch. d'Ophtal.* **42**, 321.
1928. DEUTSCHMANN, F. *Klin. Monatsbl. f. Augenheilk.* **80**, 531.
1929. —— *Arch. f. Ophthal.* **122**, 359.

THE THEORY OF DEPRESSION

1928-9. BAURMANN, M. *Klin. Monatsbl. f. Augenheilk.* **80**, 682.
1929. DE DECKER, J. F. *Arch. f. Augenheilk.* **100-1**, 180.

THE INCIDENCE OF LOW TENSION

1919. KÜMMELL, R. *Klin. Monatsbl. f. Augenheilk.* **65**, 405.
1920. GONIN, J. *Brit. Jl. of Ophthal.* (abstract), **4**, 287.
1921. KÜMMELL, R. *Klin. Monatsbl. f. Augenheilk.* **67**, 180.
1923. FUCHS, E. *Text-book of Ophthal.* 7th edn., 755.
1924. BAURMANN, M. *Arch. f. Ophthal.* **122**, 415.
1924. —— *Ber. über d. deutsch. ophthal. Gesell.*
1925. THOMAS. *Zeitschr. f. Augenheilk.* **54**, 333.

1926. HALBERTSMA, K. *Klin. Monatsbl. f. Augenheilk.* **77**, 86.
1927. GALLOIS, J. *Bull. Soc. d'ophtal. de Paris*, Feb. 106.
1928. SEDAN, J. *Ibid.* Dec. 574.

THE CAUSES OF LOW TENSION

1876. SCHNABEL. *Arch. f. Augenheilk.* **5**, 67.
1908. LAUBER, H. *Zeitschr. f. Augenheilk.* **20**, 118, 208.
1916. LEBER, TH. *Die Krankheiten der Netzhaut*, Leipzig, 1422.
1921. KILLICK, C. *Brit. Jl. of Ophthal.* **5**, 54.
1924. WEEKERS, L. *Bull. Soc. belge d'Ophtal.* 43.
1924. LEPLAT, G. *Ann. d'Ocul.* **161**, 87.
1924. VOGT, A. *Klin. Monatsbl. f. Augenheilk.* **72**, 212.
1928. MELLER, J. *Arch. of Ophthal.* **57**, 134.
1929. MAGITOT, A. *Ann. d'Ocul.* **166**, 356 ff.
1929. FRY, W. E. *Amer. Jl. of Ophthal.* **12**, 586.
1929. BEIGELMAN, M. *Arch. of Ophthal.* **1**, 463.

THE EFFECTS OF LOW TENSION AND DETACHMENT OF THE CHOROID

1917. PLOCHER, R. P. *Klin. Monatsbl. f. Augenheilk.* **59**, 610.
1921. FRANK, E. *Ibid.* **64**, 143.
1921. GUIST, G. G. *Zeitschr. f. Augenheilk.* **45**, 61.
1921. FUCHS, E. *Arch. f. Ophthal.* **104**, 468.
1922. ELLIOT, R. H. *A Treatise on Glaucoma*, London, 2nd edn., 591.
1923. ZUR NEDDEN. *Meller's Ophthalmic Surgery.* Trans. by Sweet, 317.
1924. FUCHS and KALT. *Arch. d'Ophtal.* **41**, 501.
1930. FUCHS, E. *Arch. of Ophthal.* **3**, 419.

HYPOTONY IN DIABETIC COMA

1904. KRAUSE. *Verhandl. d. Kong. finn. Med.* **21**, 439.
1906. HEINE, L. *Klin. Monatsbl. f. Augenheilk.* **44**, 2, 451.
1915. HERTEL. *Arch. f. Ophthal.* **90**.
1916. REISMAN. *Jl. Amer. Med. Assoc.* **66**, 85.
1921. WAGENER, H. P. and WILDER, R. M. *Ibid.* **76**, 515.
1923. MIDDLETON, W. S. *Wisconsin Med. Jl.* **21**, 458.
1924. GALLUS. *Klin. Monatsbl. f. Augenheilk.* **73**, 491.
1924. GIFFO. *Med. Press* (26th March), 260.
1925. ASCHER, K. W. *Ber. über d. deutsch. Ophthal. Gesell.* 186.
1925. MARX, E. *Nederl. Tijdschr. v. Geneesk.* **2**, 918.
1925. —— *Jl. Amer. Med. Assoc.* (abstract), **85**, 1265.
1925. VERHOEFF, F. H. and WAITE, J. H. *Trans. Amer. Ophthal. Soc.* 120.
1926. RICHTER, A. *Klin. Monatsbl. f. Augenheilk.* **76**, 835.
1927. BOWEN and KOENIG. *Buffalo Gen. Hosp. Bull.* **51**, 31.
1928. MCBEAN, G. M. *Amer. Jl. of Ophthal.* **11**, 825.
1928. JOSLIN, E. P. *Treatment of Diabetes Mellitus*, 4th edn., Philadelphia, 173, 658.

1929. PATEK, A. J. *Jl. Amer. Med. Assoc.* 9th Feb. **92**, 438.
1929. ALPERIN, D. *Amer. Jl. of Ophthal.* **12**, 486.
1929. VESTERGAARD, J. D. E. *Acta ophthal.* **7**, 273.

TRANSUDATE OR INFLAMMATORY EXUDATE

1920. VAIL, D. T. *Arch. of Ophthal.* **49**, 553.
1921. SHAHAN, W. E. *Amer. Jl. of Ophthal.* **4**, 108.
1921. KÜMMELL, R. *Klin. Monatsbl. f. Augenheilk.* **67**, 180.
1922. WESSELY, K. *Ibid.* **68**, 275.
1924. CURRAN, E. J. *Brit. Jl. of Ophthal.* **8**, 414.
1924. WEEKERS, L. *Bull. Soc. belge d'Ophtal.* **43**.
1924. KÜMMELL, R. *Klin. Monatsbl. f. Augenheilk.* **73**, 776.
1925. WEEKERS, L. *Arch. d'Ophtal.* June, 327.
1925. CURRAN, E. J. *Arch. of Ophthal.* **54**, 321.
1925 a. KÜMMELL, R. *Arch. f. Augenheilk.* **95**.
1925 b. —— *Klin. Monatsbl. f. Augenheilk.* **74**, 824.
1928. —— *Ibid.* **80**, 531.
1929. BAURMANN, M. *Arch. f. Ophthal.* **122**, 415.

THE THEORY OF EXUDATION

1873. STEFFAN. *Jahresber. über Verwalt. Med. Frankfurt.* **17**, 18.
1893. SCHERL. *Arch. f. Augenheilk.* **28**, 526.
1895. TEILLAIS. *Recueil d'Ophtal.* 622.
1920. FRENKEL, H. *Rev. gén. d'Ophtal.* **34**, 1.
1920. FUCHS, E. *Arch. de Oftal. Hisp. Amer.* **20**, 293.
1921. KÜMMELL, R. *Klin. Monatsbl. f. Augenheilk.* **67**, 180.
1921. MASUDA, T. *Amer. Jl. of Ophthal.* **4**, 311.
1922. CASSIDY, W. A. and GIFFORD, S. R. *Amer. Jl. of Ophthal.* **5**, 434.
1922. ORLANDINI. *Ann. di Ottal.* 445.
1923. STANKA, R. *Klin. Monatsbl. f. Augenheilk.* **70**, 707.
1923. GOURFEIN-WELT, L. *Ibid.* **70**, 565.
1923. SEGI. *Ibid.* **71**, 53.
1925. WEEKERS, L. *Arch. d'Ophtal.* June, **40**, 327.
1926. TEN DOESCHATE. *Klin. Monatsbl. f. Augenheilk.* **76**, 139.
1927. FRIEDENWALD, J. S. *Bull. Johns Hopkins Hosp.* **40**, 201.
1929. —— *Arch. of Ophthal.* May, 575.
1930. REICHLING. *Klin. Monatsbl. f. Augenheilk.* **84**, 118.

ASSOCIATION WITH NEPHRITIS

1855. V. GRAEFE, A. *Arch. f. Ophthal.* **2**, 202.
1911. VERDERAME, P. *Klin. Monatsbl. f. Augenheilk.* **49**, 452.
1921. OCHI, S. *Nippon Gank. Zasshi.* July,
1924. HILL, E. *Arch. of Ophthal.* **53**, 157.

1925. MOORE, R. FOSTER. *Medical Ophthalmology*, 2nd edn., London, 189.
1929. HANSSEN, R. *Klin. Monatsbl. f. Augenheilk.* **82**, 40.
1929. FRY, W. E. *Arch. of Ophthal.* **1**, 609
1930. FUCHS, A. *Klin. Monatsbl. f. Augenheilk.* **84**, 39.

ASSOCIATION WITH INFLAMMATION

1854. v. GRAEFE, A. *Arch. f. Ophthal.* **1**.
1903. TERSON, A. *Bull. Soc. franç. d'Ophtal.* 209.
1910. DOR, L. *Ibid.* 224.
1913. v. HIPPEL, E. *Ber. über die Vers. d. deutsch. der ophth. Ges.* **39**, 385.
1920. SCHREIBER, L. *Arch. f. Ophthal.* **103**, 750.
1920. MARTIN AMAT, M. *Arch. de Oftal. Hisp. Amer.* **20**, 172.
1921. VOGT, A. *Klin. Monatsbl. f. Augenheilk.* **66**, 321.
1922. BARRENECHEA, M. J. *Rev. Cubana de Oftal.* **4**, 62.
1922. BECKER, J. *Klin. Monatsbl. f. Augenheilk.* **68**, 240.
1922. CRAMER. *Ibid.* **68**, 240.
1922. HEINE, L. *Ber. über d. deutsch. ophthal. Gesell.* discussion, 25.
1922. SCHREIBER, L. *Zeitschr. f. Augenheilk.* **48**, 171.
1922. SCHALL. *Klin. Monatsbl. f. Augenheilk.* **68**, 236.
1924. HEINE, L. *Ibid.* **72**, 305.
1925. GIESLER, C. M. *Ibid.* **74**, 776.
1925. PICHLER. *Wiener. med. Wochenschr.* **75**, 2544.
1925. SOMOGYI. *Klin. Monatsbl. f. Augenheilk.* **75**, 518.
1925. ALGAN and COULET. *Bull. Soc. d'Ophtal. de Paris*, July, 336.
1926. LOWENSTEIN, A. *Arch. f. Ophthal.* **117**, 130.
1928. HEINE, L. *Klin. Monatsbl. f. Augenheilk.* **81**, 531.
1929. GREEFF, R. *Arch. f. Augenheilk.* **100-1**, 116.

SECONDARY RETINITIS

1916. LEBER, TH. *Graefe-Saemisch Handb.* 2nd edn., 7, **2**, 10, 1487.
1917. VOGT, A. *Klin. Monatsbl. f. Augenheilk.* **59**, 157.
1920. BOCKAERT. *Ber. über d. deutsch. ophthal. Gesell.*
1920. SIEGRIST, A. *Ibid.*
1921. GOURFEIN-WELT. *Rev. gén. d'Ophtal.* **35**, 387.
1921. SALZMANN. *Klin. Monatsbl. f. Augenheilk.* **66**, 528.
1921. DANCO, A. *Ibid.* **67**, 87.
1921. LIPPMANN, W. *Ibid.* **67**, 63.
1921. AYKAI. *Ibid.* **66**, 951.
1921. SALZMANN, M. *Vienna Ophthal. Cong.* 416.
1923. LEEMAN. *Arch. f. Ophthal.* **112**, 152.
1923. REA, LINDSAY. *Proc. Roy. Soc. Med. Sect. Ophthal. London*, Jan.
1924. WEEKERS, L. *Jl. de Neurol. et de Psychiat.* Dec.
1924. LEPLAT, G. *Ann. d'Ocul.* 87.
1927. WEISNER, M. *Klin. Monatsbl. f. Augenheilk.* **78**, 153.

1928. PASCHEFF, C. *Ber. über d. deutsch. ophthal. Gesell.* 315.
1929. REESE, W. S. *Amer. Jl. of Ophthal.* **12**, 503.
1929. BROWN, O. H. and BARLOW, C. L. *Southwestern Med.* **13**, 507.
1930. KLEIBER, G. *Klin. Monatsbl. f. Augenheilk.* **84**, 117.

INFLUENCE OF LIGHT AND HEAT

1904. BIRCH-HIRSCHFELD. *Arch. f. Ophthal.* **58**, 469.
1920. JESS, A. *Klin. Monatsbl. f. Augenheilk.* **64**, 203.
1922. HARMAN, N. BISHOP and MACDONALD. *Brit. Med. Jl.* 637.
1927. RAUH, F. *Zeitschr. f. Augenheilk.* **64**, 48.
1929. DUKE-ELDER, W. S. and P. M. *Brit. Jl. of Ophthal.* **13**, 1.
1929. ROY, J. N. *Ibid.* **13**, 490.
1929. AMSLER, MARC. *Ann. d'Ocul.* **166**, 871.
1929. CZERNY. *Ibid.* **35**, 252.

EXPERIMENTAL WORK

1922. WESSELY, K. *Klin. Monatsbl. f. Augenheilk.* **68**, 275.
1924. WEEKERS, L. *Bull. Soc. belge d'Ophtal.* 43.

SUMMARY

1930 a. VOGT, A. *Klin. Monatsbl. f. Augenheilk.* **84**, March, illustration 26.
1930 b. *Ibid.* Illustration 4.
1930 c. *Ibid.* Illustrations 3, 26, 33.

CHAPTER IV

DIFFERENTIAL DIAGNOSIS

It is not always easy to decide whether a retinal detachment is present or not. Irregular astigmatism or the presence of opacities in the media may lead to a distortion of the fundus which closely resembles a detachment (Brazil, 1920). The discovery of a detachment, if shallow and peripheral, is often only made with difficulty. Rarely choroidal or retinal tuberculosis or syphilis may cause confusion. In the former the patient is usually young, and smaller secondary tubercles often appear elsewhere in the choroid. Evans (1922), Ginzburg (1918), Harbridge (1924), Finnoff (1929), Charles (1919), and Guzman (1922), have reported difficulty in establishing a diagnosis of tuberculosis. A circumscribed chorioretinitis, usually of syphilitic origin, may closely simulate a detachment (McCaw, 1921; Knapp, 1921). In a patient reported by the last-named, the condition was bilateral, and in the lower fundus of each eye there was a separate detachment. The whole condition cleared up on anti-syphilitic treatment. At other times masses appear in the retina due to inflammatory conditions associated with other infections or septic foci (Blair and others, 1922; Fisher, 1921). Fisher, when reporting a detachment almost certainly due to inflammatory exudate, observed that it " did not seem to float freely, but it was unlike a growth". This characteristic may aid us in distinguishing a detachment due to haemorrhage, exudate or a tumour from the ordinary idiopathic type. The difficulty in diagnosis is well shown by a patient reported by Bickerton (1924). A macular tumour had been present in an only eye for at least two years. During a year of observation no change in the size of the tumour or the central scotoma was noticed.

A retinal cyst may project into the vitreous, and as it may be covered with retinal vessels it can closely simulate a detachment (Danis, 1921). This, however, is a very rare finding. Cysts are more frequently due to degeneration after inflammation, detachment or glaucoma, than as actual causes of detachment. Cystoid degeneration, however, according to Gonin and Hanssen, acts as a cause. Fuchs (1921), when reviewing ninety-nine retinal cysts, classified them as follows: those on the outer retinal surface resulting from areas of inflammation in the retina and choroid, those on the inner surface due to traction by shrinking vitreous bands, those due to the contraction of preretinal membranes, and those associated with glaucoma or choroidal tumours.

Occasionally, after vitreous haemorrhages, it is quite difficult to decide whether the retina is actually detached. However, treatment is in vain if a detachment is due to this cause, or the result of proliferating retinitis. The possibility of a decolorised preretinal haemorrhage resembling a detachment is raised by an interesting report by Law (1928).

The retina may be detached in such gross disorders as Coats's disease (Hanssen, 1920; Crigler, 1920; Knapp, 1919; Hata, 1921; Rados, 1921), angiomatosis (Scarlett, 1925; Brandt, 1921; Erggelet, 1920), miliary aneurysms (Hata, 1921; Miyashita, 1921), and renal retinitis, or in the presence of a foreign body, or some entozoon. The history and the other fundus changes in these conditions make the differentiation from the simpler or serous type of detachment of the retina easy.

EXUDATIVE MACULAR DEGENERATION. Feingold, Coppez and Danis, and more recently Holloway and Verhoeff (1929), have described an exudative form of senile macular retinitis. De Schweinitz in his classification of macular lesions mentions a corresponding group. Often the earliest fundus change is preceded by a central scotoma, and so a diagnosis of retrobulbar neuritis may be made. Later, when a mass appears, the differentiation from sarcoma may be very difficult. The value of direct scleral transillumination in such cases is undecided. Elschnig (1919), after histological examination, concluded that the condition was a chronic degenerative process, due to primary arterio-sclerosis of the ciliary and choroidal vessels. Newly formed vessels had appeared in the centre of the mass, and its edges had become pigmented. The frequent association of a circinate type of exudate with this macular pseudo-tumour is an aid in diagnosis. In this condition, and in retinitis circinata, the earliest signs may be retinal haemorrhages. Possibly the main aetiological factor is degeneration of the fine vessels in the nerve-fibre layer in the central retinal area. Other observers consider that the initial cause is a degeneration of the chorio-capillaris, and that a transudate through the lamina vitrea occurs (Behr, 1929). Behr describes an eye with this condition which was enucleated because the mass was diagnosed as sarcoma.

RETINAL PARASITES. The common occurrence of parasites, especially in certain countries, may be seen by the numerous reports of retinal cysticercus and echinococcus (Vollaro, 1928; Silva, 1928; Carsten, 1926; Schwarzkopf, 1922; Kirschmann, 1923; Bardelli, 1923; Verwey, 1923; Wood, 1922; Biancini, 1923; Pincus, 1924; Schall, 1924; Kostitch, 1925; Golowin, 1925; Derkac, 1925; Pillat, 1920; Gallemaerts, 1926; Uhthoff, 1920; Mullen, 1920; Cramer, 1919; Santos Fernandez, 1920; Brav, 1922). In the last few years ophthalmomyiasis affecting the retina has been reported by Purtscher (1924), Zeeman (1926), Behr (1920). In all these conditions there are usually other fundus changes, or positive reactions to more or less specific tests, which facilitate the diagnosis.

CHOROIDAL SARCOMA. There is one condition, however, which is common and which at times causes the greatest difficulty in diagnosis. A choroidal sarcoma may simulate a simple detachment closely. Often the vision of the affected eye is good, and the patient young and most unwilling to sacrifice the eye. The malignancy of the tumour, moreover, makes action imperative.

The lamina vitrea which develops before any pigment is formed appears to be an effective barrier between the choroid and the retinal pigment epithelium. It resists up to a point the spread inwards even of a sarcoma. Once this resistance is overcome, the growth can extend freely and an extensive detachment soon appears. The following points in the appearance of this detachment help us to distinguish it from the simple form.

As a rule a detachment due to tumour has a more solid appearance and is less apt to be tremulous. Later, however, when an effusion has led to a more extensive detachment, the difficulty in diagnosis is greater. A tumour usually rises abruptly from the surrounding fundus. Its surface is rarely undulating or thrown into waves. As long as the displaced retina is in contact with the tumour, its surface will vary with that of the tumour. In a series of twenty eyes Lindahl (1920) was able to prove that, regardless of the extent of the detachment due to effusion, the retina was directly in contact with the most prominent parts of the tumour. He found this relationship, even though the growth was minute and the associated detachment almost complete. The retina overlying the tumour itself may show a yellow or yellowish brown colour. Later, when detachment is more extensive, a yellow colour due to a special form of subretinal fluid may appear. Lohlein considers that at times this colour may be due to blood, and may appear when a haemorrhage occurs under a simple detachment. Safar (1930), when writing of a yellowish colour which develops after haemorrhages into the anterior chamber, stated that the characteristic hue was due to a fatty degeneration. He found that the cells contained material resembling fat and a substance containing iron derived only from blood. Fuchs considers that it is simply due to retinal pigment and fatty degeneration. Rönne, however, upholds the views of the Danish school, who consider this colour to be a constant sign of sarcoma, and as rarely due to any other condition. He considers it due to the very albuminous subretinal fluid, peculiar to choroidal sarcomata. It was the only positive sign in a case reported by him until, by diascleral ophthalmoscopy, he observed a very faint lack of translucency. This eye was found to contain a sarcoma, scarcely pigmented, and of the flat variety, a type examples of which, almost without exception, are diagnosed only with the onset of glaucoma. Jaensch (1926) described an eye which was removed for glaucoma, and which, on section, was found to contain a flat sarcoma 2 mm. thick. The entire choroid was infiltrated and extensions were found in the optic nerve, through the sclera, along the vessels and nerves and in the orbit. In one eye pigmentary changes similar to those of retinitis pigmentosa were considered to be due to circulatory disturbances. They were found, however, to be due to a flat sarcoma, which involved chiefly the external choroidal layers (Archangelsky, 1925). This type of sarcoma has been confused with tuberculous choroiditis (Evans, 1922; Harbridge, 1924).

Morax (1925) has found that a slight temporary obscuration of vision, or some field defect, is often the earliest symptom. Teuilères (1926) in an instructive paper describes micropsia and failing colour vision, alteration of refraction, e.g. from + 1·25 D.S. to + 6·0 D.S. in one year, or from 1·5 D.Cyl. of astigmatism to 3·0 D.Cyl. in a month following slight injury, and the seeing of bright and coloured lights from retinal oedema due to the interference from a congested and swollen choroid. He describes cases which were at first diagnosed as simple detachment of the retina, tobacco amblyopia, and glaucoma, but, in these later, on excision, sarcomata were found. The possibility of error in diagnosis of such tumours is further shown by a patient reported by St Martin (1926). The vision of one of his patients was reduced to 6/10, and for nine months the fundus remained normal. Then a detachment of the retina with retinal haemorrhages appeared. Melanosarcoma was found, and death from liver metastases followed five years later.

Sometimes newly formed vessels may be seen on the surface of a detached retina. When the venous exit through the adjacent vasa vorticosa is interfered with, the anterior ciliary veins in the corresponding area may be distended. Chemosis was found by ten Thije (1928). Handmann (1922) found vessels in the sector of the iris, corresponding to the site of a choroidal sarcoma. Occasionally a sarcoma, starting in the outer choroidal layers, produces necrosis and inflammation of the overlying sclera and the adjacent extra-ocular muscle. An appearance of scleritis and the complaint of diplopia may be the first indications of disease (Purtscher, 1929). Elliot (1922) refers to the occurrence of corneal rupture with free haemorrhage as a result of the raised tension due to choroidal sarcoma. A diagnosis of haemorrhagic glaucoma is then probable in a patient with an extensive

PLATE VI

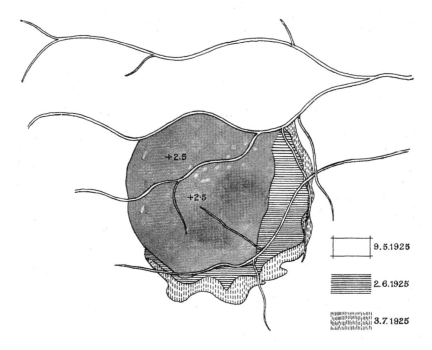

Diagrammatic representation of alteration of detachment due to a minute choroidal sarcoma. The white spots became more numerous and the dark area more prominent as time advanced.

melanotic sarcoma originating in the ciliary region. Marin Amat found the corresponding corneal quadrant to be anaesthetic (1925). Meesmann (1920) has found the slit-lamp of definite value in examining a choroidal melanosarcoma. He later confirmed by microscopical examination the appearance he had seen, viz. nodular structure and spots of pigment. Only with the narrow intense beam of the slit-lamp can one investigate the subretinal fluid. Meesmann (1927) in his atlas shows a detachment due to a small sarcoma. Vision was 5/15 and tonometry and transillumination yielded negative results. The border line between the detached area of the retina and the normal fundus was indefinite, but by means of the slit-lamp a sharp boundary was seen some distance from the edge of the detachment. On enucleation a slightly pigmented sarcoma was found surrounded by a narrow serous detachment.

Red-free light may reveal early and minute retinal haemorrhages, or the first sign of new vessel formation. It has also revealed a small detachment obscured by vitreous opacities in ordinary light (Nivault, 1920). The binocular ophthalmoscope, if the detachment lies posteriorly, often gives the best view. It reveals the transparent nature of the normal retina in a most illuminating manner. This transparence or appearance of retinal depth may be lessened, or a dark core may be seen in the centre of the detachment, if a tumour is present. No investigation of a central localised detachment is complete without an examination by these methods. By use of the slit-lamp, Elschnig (1925) was able to diagnose a cyst of the ciliary body when it had been considered a sarcoma.

A detailed drawing of such a detachment is of great value. From time to time alterations in elevation, colour or edge may appear. White spots on the surface, or areas of dark discoloration, may develop. Alterations of the inferior edge, in the cases I have watched, appeared to be most rapid. These changes are shown in Plate VI. The steady increase in size during four months led to enucleation. The tumour was 2 mm. × 1·5 mm. × 0·5 mm. Weeks described similar drawings. Much time is necessary for this, but the Zeiss drawing apparatus is of assistance. The changes are usually too fine to be revealed by photography. However, stereo-scopic photographs taken at intervals may be of value for watching more marked alterations (Bedell, 1930).

VISUAL FIELD CHANGES. The scotoma should be mapped out with minute test objects from time to time. The field defect will not be sectorial until the nerve fibres are interfered with. A gradually increasing area of blindness is very suggestive of the presence of a neoplasm, while marked variations or a scotoma which is stationary are more frequently due to other causes. Pages 123 and 124 show the alterations in a mysterious scotoma of sudden onset. The presence of a tumour was not suspected, and the fundus examination was negative. The patient disappeared for two years and nine months, and when seen again complained of intense neuralgic pain, and the eye was glaucomatous. During this period she received treatment for "nerves" and wrote stating that the eye was almost well. Therefore a persistent scotoma, especially one which tends to increase progressively in size, must be treated with great respect. After six months, the patient yielded to the severity of her pain, where persuasion had failed, and the eye was excised, revealing a melanosarcoma. Three years later this patient was still alive, and apparently well. Gourfein-Welt (1930) reports a patient with retinal haemorrhages in one eye, and a raised yellow focus close to the disc of the other eye. This fundus appearance remained unchanged for eighteen months, when suddenly an extensive detachment with raised tension appeared. After enucleation a leucosarcoma was found. From the first examination an absolute scotoma was present.

DIAGNOSTIC VALUE OF A RETINAL APERTURE. Lister (1924) holds that the presence of a hole excludes the presence of a growth. He has not seen or read of a patient in whom they existed together. He has stated that if we can detect a hole in the retina we can exclude growth, and that "if we can sub-stantiate a history of sudden loss of sight from detachment, even though a hole cannot be seen, we know that a hole must be present, and we can with equal certainty exclude growth". He supports the first statement by his experience that patho-

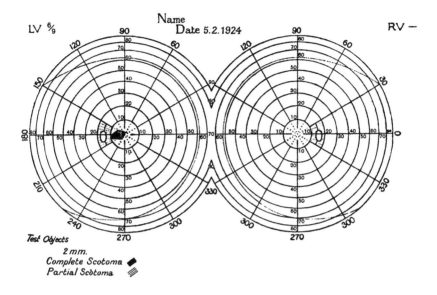

Name
Date 5.2.1924

LV 6/9   RV —

Test Objects
   2 mm.
Complete Scotoma ◆
Partial Scòtoma ⬚

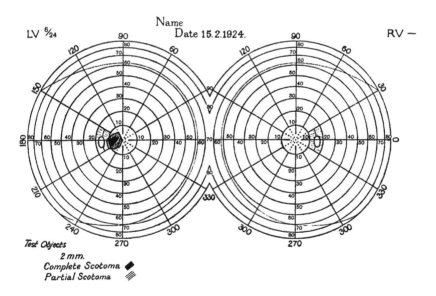

Name
Date 15.2.1924.

LV 6/24   RV —

Test Objects
   2 mm.
Complete Scotoma ◆
Partial Scotoma ⬚

Fields illustrating the scotoma caused by a choroidal sarcoma

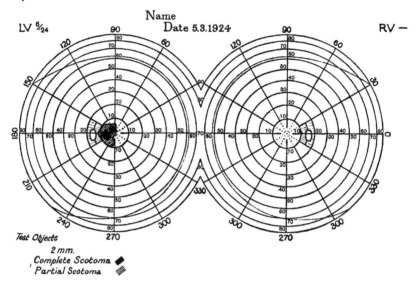

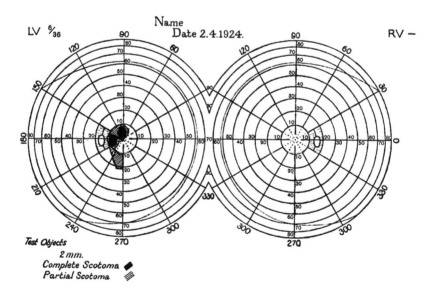

Fields illustrating the scotoma caused by a choroidal sarcoma

logical examination and clinical investigation have failed to reveal a hole where detachment was due to tumour. He finds further that in such eyes the inter-retinal fluid sets solid on fixation. This is because it has a higher albumen content than the vitreous, and, in the absence of intercommunication through a hole, it retains this. This statement has not been contradicted, and therefore we are justified in putting considerable faith in it. In the absence of other more definite signs, such as the presence of raised tension, a shadow on transillumination, new vessels, dark retinal areas on the detachment, or scleral congestion or pigmentation, the presence of a hole would justify one in being conservative.

The truth of the second statement is not so well founded. It postulates the former, and, in addition, the belief that, for the sudden development of a detachment, a hole is necessary. This point has been referred to in the section dealing with the significance of retinal tears. It is certainly not proven.

TRANSILLUMINATION. Transillumination is a method of supreme importance. Its value depends on the ability of a detached retina to transmit light and so reveal the presence of any opaque structure underlying it. Any tumour formation, even though unpigmented, will prove more or less opaque and so cast a shadow. There are several methods of transillumination, and it is well to consider them by turn.

TRANS-PUPILLARY TRANSILLUMINATION. If one wishes to investigate an anterior detachment one should focus a narrow intense beam of light, such as comes from the slit-lamp, a Lindahl lamp, or a Guist micro-arc transilluminator, through the dilated pupil (Guist, 1922). The best result is obtained if the tip of the instrument touches the cornea and the eye is rotated away from the area of the retina which one wishes to examine. By overloading the Lange scleral lamp, one gets an excellent result. The normal picture to be seen depends on the varied degree of pigmentation of the tissues through which the light passes. In a red field one will see a dark ring due to the ora serrata. From it a series of dark radially placed projections run a varying distance forwards into a weakly illuminated area corresponding to the orbiculus ciliaris. Anterior to this lies a diffuse shadow due to the ciliary body. Immediately posterior to the ora serrata the choroid appears to be more translucent than elsewhere. One may at times see a brightly illuminated stripe which corresponds with a long ciliary artery. Occasionally in darkly pigmented patients the orbiculus ciliaris does not transmit more light than the ora serrata and the ciliary body and the corresponding area is revealed as a single broad dark band. In children the ciliary body is broader and very dark, and the ora serrata, if it appears at all, shows simply as a fine line lying posteriorly to the dark ring which lies in the orbicular space. This ring shows few if any of the radial projections seen in the adult. The presence of a cataract or a vitreous haemorrhage only slightly affects the results of this method of transillumination. The ciliary region is separated from the cornea by a translucent zone which is widest in youth and whenever the anterior chamber is deep, and narrowest in the senile, especially if the angle is shallow. This clear area is normally 1·5 to 2 mm. wide. The iris may become transparent. Any pigmented tumour will interfere with the translucence of the ocular coats and will cause a shadow.

TRANSCONJUNCTIVAL METHODS. One may supplement this method by applying one of the various transilluminators to the conjunctiva. This method can be called the ordinary or the transconjunctival method, to distinguish it from a method to be described later, the trans-scleral method. Any of the instruments provided for this purpose are suitable if the light is intense, and transmitting tube or cone is opaque so that lateral scattering of the light is reduced to a minimum. By suitable rotation of the eye a considerable area can be explored in this way. The lamps of Guist (1922), Lange (1906), Lindahl (1914, 1920) and of Dalen (1925) are probably the best for this examination. One must not confuse the normal shadows due to the ciliary region with those due to pathological conditions. It is necessary to make sure that the tip of the transilluminator is posterior to this region before considering any shadow to be due to a tumour. The greatest help is obtained by always transilluminating the normal eye first.

PLATE VII

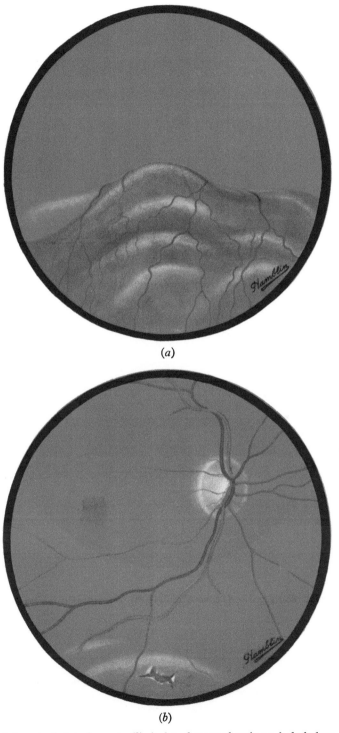

(a)

(b)

(a) A retinal detachment. (b) A detachment showing a hole below.

The translucence of the coats of the eye can be studied in two ways—the indirect and the direct method. For the indirect method, one applies the lamp to the globe, and studies the pupillary reflex. The best results are given if the light is not intense, but just sufficient to reveal the normal red reflex. When the tip of the transilluminator lies over any opaque area, a shadow will be cast which will blot out this reflex. For the direct method one uses a stronger light and, with one's eye very close, looks through the fully dilated pupil. One will see the retinal vessels, and if a tumour is pre-equatorial, its shadow may be seen. Lindahl has found this direct examination of value in finding perforating wounds or scars. They are recognised as brightly illuminated areas and a retained foreign body shows as a dark spot. One can study the fundus with the ophthalmoscope and so focus with the necessary lenses.

This method is best suited for patients with prominent eyes and those that are only lightly pigmented. The presence of the brow and bridge of the nose make it difficult to transilluminate behind the superior and the nasal ciliary regions. To study the lower half of the globe one can either apply the instrument temporally and inspect the sclera on the same side, or one can insert the instrument under the upper orbital margin and study the sclera on the opposite side of the eye. At times the normal ciliary region is so opaque that the transmitted light is insufficient to illuminate the pupil and give a reflex. This is most apt to cause trouble if one wishes to transilluminate the upper choroid in a patient who has deep-set eyes or a difficulty in downward rotation. One must take into consideration the effects of varying pigmentation. It is wise always to transilluminate the normal eye first. In using a Lange lamp one must apply the tip accurately for the incident and therefore the transmitted light will vary accordingly.

TRANS-SCLERAL METHOD. If the tumour is situated posteriorly, especially if it lies close to the macula or disc, the former method may be used. But the method of choice is the direct trans-scleral. One incises the conjunctiva and the capsule of

Tenon, and passes the sterilised tip of a Lange, a Lancaster (1913) or a Dalen lamp round the eye until it is opposite the area under consideration. It is essential that the room be dark, that one should apply the tip of the lamp accurately, and that one's eye be close to the patient's cornea. The more one keeps extraneous light from entering one's eye the better one is able to study the effects of transillumination, no matter which method is being used. Apart from the clear view of the retinal vessels, and of any other feature present, one sees a pink light shining through the porus opticus. If a simple detachment is present, it will appear red, and the vessels black, even though the retina appears grey by the ophthalmoscope. The normal area of the fundus will appear dark and so there is a much greater contrast between the normal and the detached areas of retina by this method than by ophthalmoscopy. A tumour will interfere with the translucence of the retina in a manner which will vary with the degree of pigmentation. If the retina lies at a considerable distance from the choroid, one requires a light of greater intensity. For such detachments, Fuchs uses a glass cone which fits on to Hess's hammer lamp. In one eye in which the difference in level was 10 D., he obtained a good shadow by this method. It is sometimes wise to vary the intensity of the light. Alternate examination with the transilluminator and a luminous ophthalmoscope is most instructive. An assistant can switch the light of the former instrument on or off as required (Erggelet). The comparison of the two views has been of great help. Once by this combined method the only shadows visible were those due to three macular haemorrhages visible by ophthalmoscopy. So transillumination was considered negative. On other advice the eye was removed, and no neoplasm was present. Lindahl (1920) reported three retinal detachments which gave definite findings when examined by these two methods, and which were found to be due to tumours.

Ophthalmoscopic transillumination which is often neglected, but the value of which has been emphasised by Lindahl (1920), is a simple and at times a useful method. If one uses an electric lamp with a concentrated and exposed filament, and examines by direct ophthalmoscopy, the light concentrated on the detached area of retina will appear as a small spot, the surrounding retina more or less red and the vessels black. If the surrounding retina appears opaque, the presence of a tumour, or possibly a haemorrhage, is proved. Gullstrand's ophthalmoscope is of special value for this investigation. In principle this method is similar to examination by the beam of the slit-lamp.

Trans-scleral transillumination is of great importance. More elaborate instruments such as Hertzell's water-cooled lamp (1908–9) for transillumination from the naso-pharynx are of much less value. Langenhans later modified this lamp and used it widely (1910). The water-cooling apparatus makes this lamp awkward to use, and it is necessary to cover the patient's face with an opaque mask to shut out extraneous light. The tip of the Lange lamp can be put within three millimetres of the macula on the temporal side, and almost as close to the disc nasally. Holth (1926), Rönne (1928), and others report eyes containing sarcomata, the presence of which would have been recognised if this method had been used, and which were undiagnosed until this method was adopted. The excellence of this method was shown in a clinical history reported by Klein (1929). The affected fundus of a female patient aged forty-four showed a detachment close to the macula. Transillumination revealed two separate shadows, and two distinct tumours were revealed on section. However, a few cases remain extraordinarily difficult to diagnose. Of these, that described by Shoemaker and De Long (1926) is a good example.

The patient, who was aged seventy-three, had noticed a gradual loss of vision in one eye for four or five months. An extensive detachment was found. In the upper inner quadrant an overhanging brownish mass was found just behind the lens. There was no movement of any portion of the detached retina. "Transillumination gave dense opacity and extensive shadow as confirmatory evidence of a solid growth." After excision even the macroscopic appearances made the diagnosis of sarcoma almost certain. However, on microscopic examination it was found that only serous

AR   9 exudate lay between the retina and the choroid. It was dark in colour and degenerate. The underlying cause was considered to be irido-cyclitis, which probably was related to an attack of pneumonia eleven months before.

The best results will be obtained if one uses Lange's lamp for examining the posterior half and either a Lindahl or a Guist transilluminator for the anterior half of the eye.

THE EXAMINATION OF THE ORA SERRATA (*v.* Plate II *b*). The problem of "total ophthalmoscopy" has been tackled by many observers in different ways. For us, now that Gonin's method of operation is pre-eminent, the ora serrata assumes an added importance. In shining a light through the sclera, and examining the fundus by means of diverse diaphanoscopes, Reuss, Rochon-Duvigneaud, Lange, Sachs and others were applying a method that A. von Graefe, in 1868, used for distinguishing scleral ectasia from episcleral and choroidal sarcomata. Hertzell (1909) and Langenhans (1910) shone a light through from the pharynx. Sachs (1903) exerted pressure on the globe with the end of his instrument, and appears to have been the first to see clearly the anterior region of the fundus.

Trantas' method is definitely of value for examining the pre-equatorial fundus. The whole fundus including the ciliary region can be examined by it. The diaphanoscope is similar to a Lange lamp, and pressure is made by its tip on the sclera at the site corresponding to the area of fundus one wishes to see. Sometimes digital pressure on the sclera is used. Pressure is unnecessary if a coloboma of the iris or a forward dislocation of the lens is present. The eye is rotated in a suitable direction. The ciliary processes can be studied if pressure is made on the limbus in the direction of the posterior pole of the lens. One examines with a loupe or + 15·0 D.S. or + 20·0 D.S. lens in the ophthalmoscope. The pupil must be fully dilated; Trantas preferring euphthalmine for this purpose. Vogt recommends digital pressure, or pressure made by an assistant with a glass rod or a Daviel spoon, for investigation of this area with the ophthalmoscope or the slit-lamp.

There is a prismatic lens (*lentille-prisme*) designed by Galezowski which is of service in exploring the ora serrata. By this the earliest degeneration in myopia was found to occur close to the ora serrata rather than close to the macula and disc (Barabaschow, 1928). By ordinary methods the anterior but not the posterior surface of the ciliary processes are visible if an iris coloboma or an anterior dislocation of the lens exists. A grey reflex may be visible in the extreme periphery. It is probably due to the periphery of the lens (Salzmann, 1921). It has been shown by means of the slit-lamp that the optical limit of the retina in eyes with refraction between + 6 and − 10 D. is about 7 mm. from the limbus. This distance is reduced by half in aphakia (Scullica, 1925). By Trantas' method one can study the uveal circulation and pigment distribution. During pressure the sclera becomes visible as the choroidal vessels empty, and then on relaxation they refill with blood. During pressure the luminosity through the disc increases. If one presses over a patch of choroidal atrophy, it loses its redness and similarity to the rest of the fundus and becomes white. The vorticose veins and the long and short ciliary arteries can be seen.

CHANGES IN TENSION. Priestley Smith (1891) found no exception to the following rule, that if an eye containing a tumour was excised while tension was still normal, the filtration angle would be found open, but that it would be found closed if excision was performed after the tension had risen. Greeves (1914) considered that not only is the growth of the tumour, especially when the detachment is total and a compensating loss of aqueous and fluid vitreous can no longer occur, a cause of raised tension, but also that there is in some eyes a mild irido-cyclitis with blockage of the pectinate ligament.

As a rule the tension of an eye containing a detachment of the retina due to a choroidal tumour becomes raised. The stage at which this occurs depends more on its site than on its size. It depends on the effect the growth has on the uveal circulation, and the resulting transudation. As a rule the period of relative tolerance of the eye to the tumour is shorter when it is situated in the ciliary or equatorial region, and more prolonged if it is on the posterior pole. At times one does not see the patient until the eye presents the picture of a typical congestive glaucoma. If such an attack is due to the presence of a tumour, failing vision will almost certainly have been noticed for some time, in contrast to the unexpected onset of primary glaucoma. In the latter, also, the other eye is rarely normal. The difficulty in distinguishing the two conditions is seen when one recalls the frequency with which a diagnosis of glaucoma has been made, and later a sarcoma has been revealed. In many of these an operation has been done for the purpose of reducing tension. This difficulty is emphasised by the numerous reports made in the last few years: Guion and Berens (1924), Aurand (1925), Muirhead (1922), Ellett (1920), May and Williamson-Noble (1922), Maxey (1923), Williamson-Noble (1925), Jaensch (1926), Friedenwald (1926), Peters (1921), Cross (1922), Fileti (1925), Cayce (1925), Brawley (1925), Schwartz (1925), Stieren (1925).

Tension may be raised in retinal detachment even though no neoplasm is present. It may be a rare finding, but if eyes are examined soon after the onset it will be found more frequently than Thomas found it in a series of 247 patients, namely once (1925). If raised tension is found it is usually because the retina is pushed forwards by haemorrhage (Bergmeister, 1919) or exudate (Raeder, 1925). In two young female patients with raised tension and retinal detachment a diagnosis of sarcoma was made. Enucleation, however, revealed irido-cyclitis only (Morax, 1920). The association of raised tension and detachment was found in glaucoma, exudative choroiditis and after haemorrhages by Joltrois (1924). Maggiore (1923) reported five eyes which were myopic and showed a detachment with raised tension. On histological examination plastic iritis and choroiditis were found. Elliot (1922) quoted Nordenson's series of 126 eyes with spontaneous detachments in which six had raised tension. Three of these eyes showed signs of irido-cyclitis. He also refers to Keukenschryver's thesis (1916) in which five similar eyes were described. He believes that, as a result of retinal degeneration, especially in high myopia, irritant substances are liberated which produce a uveitis and a subsequent obstruction at the angle of the anterior chamber. It is interesting to realise that if secondary glaucoma develops in the course of a detachment, the detachment may grow less (Sedan, 1928).

Fuchs (1920) finds that there are three main ways in which glaucoma can be associated with detachment. Either glaucoma, primary or secondary, may cause the detachment, or the detachment may cause the glaucoma, or both may be due to the same agent, as in retinal thrombosis. In other eyes the exact mechanism eludes discovery. If the raised tension is not due to the effusion of fluid or a haemorrhage, it may be due to the obstruction of Schlemm's canal by substances formed in the neighbourhood of the detachment.

Terrien (1926) refers to eleven patients of whom he knew, from whom unsuspected eyes were removed, and the subsequent finding of a tumour was made. Neame and Wajid Ali Khan (1925), when investigating the 402 blind painful eyes removed at Moorfields during a period of eleven years, found that forty contained choroidal sarcoma, and that, of these, there had been no suspicion of it in at least sixteen. The finding of sarcoma in 10 per cent. of such a series is further proof that the only proper treatment for blind painful eyes with raised tension is excision. The presence of a tumour may be expected if after an iridectomy the wound fails to heal, or if recurrent haemorrhages occur from the iris. Blind painful glaucomatous eyes should be excised, except in the rare cases in which the fundus can be seen. There should be no need to emphasise the necessity for section of all excised eyes. If a tumour is detected the orbit should be radiated thoroughly. In the small group of blind painful eyes with transparent media, if a detachment of the retina is detected and transillumination is negative, Neame suggests the following methods of investigation:

(1) With a sharp needle, puncture the sclera opposite the detachment, and examine the fundus to see if the detachment grows less. Meisner (1923) reports five eyes, in some of which transillumination was negative, in which he did this and found sarcoma cells in the fluid drawn off. Gérard and Detroy (1926), on doing this, could draw off no fluid, so

excised the eye and found a small melanosarcoma. Esser (1924), Ballantyne (1922) and others considered this a justifiable procedure. That it is dangerous is the view of Terrien (1926) and of Scheerer and Fehr, who found a rapid extension of the growth under the conjunctiva to the site of the puncture. Archangelsky (1929) reports that he has found this method of no value. It is therefore a procedure rarely justifiable, and then only if transillumination has failed, and if one is prepared to enucleate immediately. Valuable time may be lost if one puts confidence in a negative result. Burton Chance (1926) emphatically expressed similar views.

(2) The dissection of a scleral flap with its apex placed anteriorly, over the site of detachment. The flap should be cautiously raised so as not to damage a tumour if present.

MISLEADING SIGNS. A detached retina due to a choroidal sarcoma may also be camouflaged by the development of irido-cyclitis. This is due to necrotic changes in the tumour. Many eyes have been removed for cyclitis or panophthalmitis or even sympathetic ophthalmitis, with or without raised tension, and sarcoma revealed after section of the eye (Rollet and Bussy, 1923; Butler and Assinder, 1924; Cohen, 1924–5; Michael, 1924; Peterfi, 1925; Fuchs, 1921; Redaelli, 1922; Velhagen, 1922; Schwartz, 1927). Marin Amat's patient (1924) was a girl aged nine, whose eye was removed for panophthalmitis, and eight months later the orbit was full of a recurrence of tumour, which was found to be glioma. Terrien (1926) describes a series of old shrunken eyes which on excision were found to contain sarcomata. A man aged fifty-four had an eye which had been atrophic all his life. It became painful and was excised, and a sarcoma was found. In another patient reported by Terrien, the picture was that of advanced irido-cyclitis, with unusually severe pain. Tension was not raised. On section the anterior half of the eye revealed irido-cyclitis and the posterior half a leucosarcoma. The possible confusion with irido-cyclitis is so great that it led Mawas (1924) to write an article entitled "Sarcoma infectieux de l'œil humain".

Unfortunately one cannot rely on the presence of raised tension as a certain sign of tumour. Necrotic changes or irido-cyclitis may explain the occasional occurrence of choroidal sarcoma with low tension. Green (1920), Francis (1920), Griscom (1923), Heine (1923) and others have described such instances. In Heine's patient a choroidal sarcoma had perforated the retina and so lowered the tension. In a series of twelve patients Heymans (1921) found four with reduced tension. The association of detachment of the retina and raised tension occurs earlier when tumours are near the ciliary region than when situated posteriorly (Koliopoulos, 1929). The possibility of this association of low tension with detachment due to tumour formation must be kept in mind if an early diagnosis is to be made.

Many have described the absence of a shadow on transillumination in an eye in which later a sarcoma, usually a leucosarcoma, was found. Rowan (1923) and Doesschate (1921) have described eyes which were negative on transillumination and had low tension, and yet developed melanosarcoma. Levy (1922) described a fundus which was clear at first, and ten months later showed a dark shadow. On excision, a partially pigmented tumour was found. Seefelder (1926) reported a retrochoroidal haemorrhage and Shoemaker (1926) a choroidal exudate which simulated sarcoma by casting shadows. Treacher Collins (1920) reported a translucent tumour of the ciliary body which proved to be a leucosarcoma. As Neame (1920) has remarked, "A cyst containing blood pigment may cast a shadow, while a tumour free of pigment may be translucent". If the detached retina is a certain distance from the tumour its shadow may not be seen. These cases fortunately are not common and, as Holth (1926) remarks, improved technique and the wider use of more up-to-date lamps will greatly lessen this difficulty.

In differentiating simple detachments of the retina from those due to tumour, one can sometimes get assistance from the method of onset. A vitreous haemorrhage or the appearance of retinal haemorrhages may herald the advance of a choroidal sarcoma (Rönne, 1923). Occasionally a choroidal sarcoma will adhere to the retina, perforate it with a minimum of detachment and spread through into the vitreous. The first symptom is usually sudden blindness, due to vitreous haemorrhage. As the blood clears, a spherical mass with a greyish brown surface is seen projecting into the vitreous. It may be distinguished from a simple vitreous haemorrhage by the manner in which, in the latter, transilluminated light shines through between the opaque mass and the choroid. This reveals the fact that it lies at some distance from the choroid. It is remarkable that such a tumour can push through the retina and not necessarily produce a sectorial defect, but simply a scotoma. These tumours have usually been found to be cavernous sarcomata. Usher (1923) emphasises the fact that in the literature sarcoma was bilateral in 30 per cent. of 186 detachments. Seible found 12·3 per cent. to be bilateral. If watched over a longer period this proportion would be greater. Merkel (1926) considers the association with congenital melanosis a probable aetiological factor. He found nine such eyes on record which developed sarcoma. Reese (1925) stated that of twenty-eight cases of melanosis oculi in the literature 27 per cent. developed sarcoma. He added that all the patients were brunettes, but none were negroes. Doherty (1927, 1928) stated that 29 per cent. became malignant. He reported a negro in whom it occurred, and referred to blondes being affected. As the retinal pigment epithelium is not involved, and as choroidal sarcomata usually grow towards the retina, it has been suggested that an early sign of developing malignancy will be a disturbance of this retinal layer (Johnson, 1929). The actual relationship with melanosis is not universally accepted, but, even if it does not exist, it is wise to remember the extreme chronicity of certain malignant choroidal tumours. If this relationship does not exist it is difficult to explain the following occurrence. Twenty-seven years after a small round mass on the iris was first observed an eye was excised and sarcoma diagnosed (Chance, 1928). It appears that many of the so-called microscopic or "smallest" sarcomata of the choroid are melanomata and similar to the blue naevi of the skin.

A history of trauma is common before either simple detachment or detachment due to a choroidal sarcoma. Nitsch (1925) found that 15 per cent. of seventy-three young patients reported as having sarcoma gave a history of trauma, while in a series of Fuchs, quoted by Parsons, 11 per cent. gave a history of injury. The possible remoteness of trauma is stressed by Crigler (1922) who reports an eye, blinded by an injury thirty years before, which developed scleral nodules, and, on excision, a sarcoma was found. When investigating a series of 970 patients with sarcoma Coley (1898) could find a distinct history of trauma in 23 per cent. McFarland (1924) concluded that "in about 25 per cent. of tumours some kind of trauma precedes the actual appearance of the tumour, and may play a part in its origin by furnishing the necessary stimulus to make its cells grow, though in 75 per cent. no such influence can be found". Though many French and German writers appear to consider that a definite relationship exists, Ewing (1928) believed that "the ratio of tumours among injured persons is not above the normal incidence of such growths among the general population".

It is unlikely that a contusion can cause a sarcomatous growth; it is possible that it can initiate the development of such a growth in a predisposed part; it is certain, however, that the local spread and the dissemination of a sarcoma can be accelerated by trauma (Moretti, 1929; Bibliography). Stallard in his series of idiopathic detachments found a history of trauma in only 16 per cent. This corresponds with the findings of Fitsch and Fuchs in the series of ocular sarcomata just mentioned, and suggests that in the eye trauma plays only a small initiating part.

A simple detachment of the retina may tend to subside or even be cured spontaneously (see "Prognosis"), but a detachment due to a sarcoma does not retrogress. Degeneration and necrosis in ocular sarcomata appears to be very rare. It differs in this way from gliomata which have so often been seen to grow smaller (von Hippel, 1928). It appears that a glioma may become necrotic after destroying the retina. After invasion by connective tissue, tumour cells grow again, until they necrose and become calcified as the blood supply is cut off. This leads to the atrophy of the globe. Gamble has collected five examples. A complete list of examples of such retrogression is found in Sticherling's thesis (1927).

If there is any doubt regarding diagnosis, one must advise the patient that the danger lies not so much in the duration of the tumour's existence, as in the degree of malignancy present. Certain minute growths have been early associated with metastases, whilst extensive tumours have been free from such for years. So if early enucleation is agreed to, the patient cannot be promised freedom from metastasis, but only a considerably better chance. The mixed-cell type is supposed to produce a metastasis more rapidly than the spindle-cell types. Elschnig has suggested that some uveal sarcomata which prove rapidly fatal are probably not primary but secondary to some well-established growth elsewhere. Foster Moore (1930) has watched a choroidal sarcoma shrink after the insertion of two radon seeds (1 millicurie and 5 milli-curies respectively) filtered through (0·5 mm. platinum) directly into the growth. Time will prove whether dissemina-tion was prevented. If an only useful eye is affected, von Hippel (1922) advises radiation as long as useful vision re-mains. He reviewed 132 cases from the literature which had been followed for from five to thirty years; 28 per cent. of those operated on in the first stage, and 19 per cent. of those operated on in the second stage had metastases. These find-ings suggest that the initial malignancy of the tumour is the factor which determines prognosis. Webb-Johnson and McLeod (1924) report a patient who died eighteen years after enucleation, and refer to one who lived for twenty-four years. Dawson (1922) found metastases fourteen years and von Hippel eighteen years after enucleation. In Ellett's patient (1929) an abdominal metastasis appeared eighteen years after enucleation for loss of vision due to spindle-cell sarcoma of the choroid. The difficulty in prognosis is further emphasised by a report cited by Ellett (1930). After enuclea-tion the emissary veins of the globe were found to be filled with sarcoma cells, and yet the patient lived for thirty years, when death was due to other causes. Burton Chance (1928) reports a patient who was alive for three years after enuclea-tion of an eye, in which a tumour had been observed for a year. Hirschberg's (1919) patient was alive twenty-eight years after excision for sarcoma. This he considered the longest on record. Once a metastasis does appear it grows with extraordinary rapidity. Grosz (1929) found the mortality from proved sarcoma to be 50 per cent. For bibliography of melanotic sarcoma see Howard's article (1926).

METASTATIC CARCINOMA. Difficulty in diagnosis is less when the detachment is due to a metastatic carcinoma. Usher (1923) sums up the literature on this subject to 1922. Since then patients have been reported by Maggiore (1923), Gamble (1925), Fileti (1925), Knapp (1925), Usher (1926), Clapp (1926), Singer (1926), Pollakova (1929).

A choroidal metastasis from a chorio-epithelioma has been reported by Mulock Houwer (1926). This appears to be unique. A metastatic endothelioma is referred to by Adrogué (1924), and a metastatic spindle-celled sarcoma with the primary growth in the ovary is described by Elschnig (1926). He stated that only two other similar metastatic tumours had been reported and that in each the primary had been a naevus on the skin.

GLIOMA OR RETINO-BLASTOMA. In infants difficulty may arise in distinguishing simple detachments from gliomata, especially those due to haemorrhage. The possibility of a detachment due to haemorrhage in early life is understood when one remembers the frequency of intra-ocular haemorrhage in the new-born. Retinal haemorrhages were found in 26 per cent. of new-born infants examined as a routine by Paul, Stumpf and Sicherer (1909) and by Jacobs (1924). Lachman (1927) reported an infant whose eyes were excised because of bilateral detachment simulating glioma. In these and in eyes described by Stoewer (1907) and Rockliffe (1898) the detachment was due to haemorrhage. Leber (1926), Sattler (1926), Fernandez (1920) and Clarke (1898) have reported between them ten children with simple detachment simulating glioma.

It must not be forgotten that glioma may simulate irido-cyclitis, and enucleation be postponed. In a patient reported by Aubineau and Opin (1922) a diagnosis of tuberculous or metastatic irido-cyclitis was made. The whole problem of the differentiation of the conditions which resemble glioma is involved in such a patient. As the majority of the affected eyes are blind, and almost certain to become degenerate, enucleation is usually the wisest treatment. The occasional occurrence of sarcoma in quite young children and the occurrence of glioma at times in older ones and even in adults are facts of importance (Gérard and Detroy, 1926). It is possible that some of the "gliomata" found in the eyes of adults were really benign conditions such as massive gliosis (Friedenwald, 1926). But the growth found in the eye of a man aged forty-eight by Verhoeff (1929) was an undoubted retino-blastoma. The female patient aged twenty, reported by Maghy (1919), was found to have an extensive glioma in her only eye. The other eye had been excised eighteen years before, and had contained a similar growth.

REFERENCES

GENERAL

1918. GINZBURG, G. *Klin. Monatsbl. f Augenheilk.* **61**, 643.
1919. KNAPP, A. *Arch of Ophthal.* **48**, 559.
1919. CHARLES, J. W. *Ibid.* **48**, 569.
1920. ERGGELET, H. *Klin. Monatsbl. f. Augenheilk.* **65**, 413.
1920. HANSSEN, R. *Ibid.* **65**, 705.
1920. BRAZIL, W. H. *Trans. Ophthal. Soc. U.K.* **40**, 373.
1920. CRIGLER, L. W. *Arch. of Ophthal.* **49**, 287.
1921. FISHER, J. H. *Trans. Ophthal. Soc. U.K.* **41**, 235.
1921. DANIS, M. *Amer. Jl. of Ophthal.* (abstract), **4**, 279.
1921. FUCHS, A. *Arch. f. Ophthal.* **105**, 333.
1921. HATA. *Amer. Jl. of Ophthal.* (abstract), **4**, 306.
1921. RADOS, A. *Arch. f. Ophthal.* **105**, 973.
1921. BRANDT, R. *Ibid.* **106**, 127.
1921. MIYASHITA, S. *Brit. Jl. of Ophthal.* **5**, 448.
1921. McCAW, J. A. *Amer. Jl. of Ophthal.* **4**, 539.
1921. KNAPP, A. *Arch. of Ophthal.* **50**, 242.
1922. EVANS, J. *Trans. Ophthal. Soc. U.K.* **42**, 304.
1922. GUZMANN. *Zeitschr. f. Augenheilk.* **49**, 143.
1922. BLAIR, C. L. and others. *Amer. Jl. of Ophthal.* **5**, 217
1924. BICKERTON, H. R. *Trans. Ophthal. Soc. U.K.* **44**, 404
1924. HARBRIDGE, D. F. *Southwestern Med.* **7**, 36.
1925. SCARLETT, H. W. *Amer. Jl. of Ophthal.* **8**, 493.
1928. LAW, F. W. *Brit. Jl. of Ophthal.* **12**, 646.
1929. FINNOFF, W. C. *Ill. Med. Jl.* 198.

EXUDATIVE MACULAR DEGENERATION

1919. HOLLOWAY, T. B. and VERHOEFF, F. H. *Arch. of Ophthal.* Feb. **1**, 219.
1919. ELSCHNIG, A. *Klin. Monatsbl. f. Augenheilk.* **62**, 145, Feb.
1929. BEHR, CARL. *Zeitschr. f. Augenheilk.* **69**, 1.

The exudative form of macular degeneration is well described in
1915. *Amer. Encycl. of Ophthal.* **15**, 11, 344.
1916. *Trans. Amer. Ophthal. Soc.* **14**, 753.

RETINAL PARASITES

1919. CRAMER. *Zeitschr. f. Augenheilk.* **41**, 55.
1920. BEHR, C. *Klin. Monatsbl. f. Augenheilk.* **64**, 161.
1920. PILLAT, A. *Wein. Klin. Wochenschr.* **33**, 925.
1920. UHTHOFF, W. *Klin. Monatsbl. f. Augenheilk.* **64**, 120.
1920. MULLEN. *Texas State Jl. of Med.* **16**, 293.
1920. FERNANDEZ, J. SANTOS. *Rev. Cubana de Oftal.* **5a**, 756.
1922. SCHWARZKOPF, G. *Klin. Monatsbl. f. Augenheilk.* **68**, 632.
1922. WOOD, D. J. *Brit. Jl. of Ophthal.* **6**, 459.
1922. BRAV, A. *Eye, Ear, Nose and Throat Monthly,* **1**, 61.
1923. KIRSCHMANN. *Klin. Monatsbl. f. Augenheilk.* **70**, 557.
1923. BARDELLI, L. *Arch. d'Ophtal.* **40**, 60.
1923. VERWEY, A. *Med. Jl. South Africa,* **18**, 250.
1923. BIANCINI. *Ann. di Ottal.* **51**, 479.
1924. PURTSCHER, A. *Klin. Monatsbl. f. Augenheilk.* **72**, 764.
1924. PINCUS, F. *Münch. med. Wochenschr.* 18th Jan. 89.
1924. SCHALL, E. *Klin. Wochenschr.* Feb. 301.
1925. KOSTITCH, D. *Ann. d'Ocul.* **162**, 528.
1925. GOLOWIN, S. S. *Klin. Monatsbl. f. Augenheilk.* **75**, 842.
1925. DERKAC, V. *Zeitschr. f. Augenheilk.* **57**, 605.
1926. GALLEMAERTS, E. *Soc. d'Ophtal. de Paris,* July, 344.
1926. ZEEMAN, W. F. *Zeitschr. f. Augenheilk.* **60**, 68.
1926. CARSTEN, P. *Ibid.* **58**, 210.
1928. SILVA, R. *Amer. Jl. of Ophthal.* **2**, 869.
1928. VOLLARO, A. *Boll. d'Ocul.* **7**, 1013.

For earlier references see *Graefe-Saemisch Handbuch,* 2nd edn., 7, **2**, 10, 1922.

CHOROIDAL SARCOMA

1920. NIVAULT, P. *Retina with Red-free Light,* Paris Thesis.
1920. MEESMANN, A. *Klin. Monatsbl. f. Augenheilk.* **66**, 417.
1922. HANDMANN, M. *Ibid.* **69**, 35.
1922. ELLIOT, R. H. *A Treatise on Glaucoma,* London, 2nd edn., 379.
1924. WEEKS, J. E. *Osler Memor. Contrib. to Med. and Biolog. Research,* 1060.

1925. ELSCHNIG. *Klin. Monatsbl. f. Augenheilk.* **74**, 476.
1925. ARCHANGELSKY, W. *Ibid.* **74**, 277.
1925. MARIN AMAT, M. *Anal. de Oftal.* Sept. 521.
1925. MORAX, V. *Soc. d'Ophtal. de Paris*, Dec. 552.
1926. TEUILÈRS, M. *Arch. d'Ophtal.* July, 393.
1926. ST MARTIN. *Ann. d'Ocul.* **163**, 431.
1926. JAENSCH, P. A. *Klin. Monatsbl. f. Augenheilk.* **76**, 433.
1927. MEESMANN, A. *The Microscopy of the Living Eye with the Gullstrand Slit-lamp*, Plate 209, Berlin.
1928. TEN THIJE, P. A. *Nederl. Tijdscher. v. Geneesk*, **2**, 4321.
1929. PURTSCHER, A. *Zeitschr. f. Augenheilk.* **69**, 219.
1930. BEDELL, A. J. *Amer. Jl. of Ophthal.* **13**, 390.
1930. GOURFEIN-WELT. *Klin. Monatsbl. f. Augenheilk.* **84**, 106.
1930. SAFAR, K. *Arch. f. Ophthal.* **123**, 19.

DIAGNOSTIC VALUE OF A RETINAL HOLE

1924. LISTER, Sir WM. *Brit. Jl. of Ophthal.* **8**, 16.

TRANSILLUMINATION

1906. LANGE. *Klin. Monatsbl. f. Augenheilk.* **44**, 1.
1908–9. HERTZELL. *Berlin Klin. Wochenschr.* **45**, part 1, 11; **49**, part 2, 2097; **46**, part 2, 1892.
1910. LANGENHANS. *Ibid.* **47**, part 1, 1133.
1913. LANCASTER, W. B. *Trans. Amer. Ophthal. Soc.* **13**, 443.
1914. LINDAHL, C. *Klin. Monatsbl. f. Augenheilk.* **52**, 716.
1920. —— *Ibid.* **65**, 11.
1922. GUIST, G. *Zeitschr. f. Augenheilk.* **48**, 219.
1925. ELSCHNIG, H. H. *Klin. Monatsbl. f. Augenheilk.* **74**, 476.
1925. DALEN, A. *Ibid.* **75**, 157.
1926. HOLTH, S. *Ibid.* **76**, 510.
1926. SHOEMAKER, W. J. and DE LONG, P. *Contrib. Ophthal. Science*, Jackson vol. Wisconsin, 146.
1928. RÖNNE, H. *Ber. über d. Versamml. d. deutsch.* 241.
1929. KLEIN, N. *Klin. Monatsbl. f. Augenheilk.* **83**, 489.

THE EXAMINATION OF THE ORA SERRATA

1903. SACHS, M. *Münch. med. Wochenschr.* 742.
1909. HERTZELL. *Zeitschr. f. Augenheilk.* **21**, 185.
1910. LANGENHANS. *Ibid.* 101.
1921. SALZMANN, M. *Vienna Ophthal. Congress*, August, 416.
1921. —— *Klin. Monatsbl. f. Augenheilk.* **67**.
1925. SCULLICA. *Ann. di Ottal.* **53**, 1070.
1926. TRANTAS, A. *Arch. d'Ophtal.* **43**, 149.
1928. BARABASCHOW, P. N. *Ukrainisch Medicine Arch.* **3**.

CHANGES IN TENSION

1891. SMITH, PRIESTLEY. *Glaucoma*, London.
1914. GREEVES, R. AFFLECK. *Proc. Roy. Soc. Med.* 8th May.
1916. KEUKENSCHRYVER, N. C. Thesis, *Ophthalmology*, Amsterdam, April 1916, 533.
1919. BERGMEISTER, R. *Zeitschr. f. Augenheilk.* **42**, 254.
1920. ELLETT, E. C. *Amer. Jl. of Ophthal.* **3**, 732.
1920. MORAX, V. *Arch. d'Ophtal.* **37**, 374.
1920. FUCHS. *Arch. f. Ophthal.* **101**, 265.
1921. PETERS. *Penn. Med. Jl.* **25**, 20.
1922. MAY, H. J. and WILLIAMSON-NOBLE, F. A. *Amer. Jl. of Ophthal.* **5**, 375.
1922. MUIRHEAD, J. R. *Med. Jl. of Australia*, **2**, 720.
1922. CROSS, G. H. *Amer. Jl. of Ophthal.* Ser. 3, v. 733.
1922. BALLANTYNE, A. J. *Brit. Jl. of Ophthal.* **6**, 214.
1922. ELLIOT, R. H. *A Treatise on Glaucoma*, 2nd edn., London, 380.
1923. MAXEY, E. E. *North Western Med. Jl.* 361.
1923. MAGGIORE, L. M. *Klin. Monatsbl. f. Augenheilk.* **70**, 417.
1923. MEISNER, M. *Ibid.* **70**, 722.
1924. GUION, C. M. and BERENS, C. *Jl. Amer. Med. Assoc.* **82**, 1024.
1924. JOLTROIS. *Médecine*, **5**, 261.
1924. ESSER, F. *Klin. Monatsbl. f. Augenheilk.* **73**, 192.
1925. AURAND. *Ophthal. Year Book.* **21**.
1925. WILLIAMSON-NOBLE, F. A. *Trans. Ophthal. Soc. U.K.* **45**, 251.
1925. FILETI, A. *Ann. di Ottal.* **53**, 596.
1925. CAYCE, E. B. *Amer. Jl. of Ophthal.* **8**, 651.
1925. BRAWLEY, F. E. *Amer. Jl. of Ophthal.* Discussion, **8**, 790, 829.
1925. SCHWARTZ, V. *Ibid.* **8**, 660.
1925. STIEREN, E. *Jl. Amer. Med. Assoc.* **85**, 1213.
1925. THOMAS. *Zeitschr. f. Augenheilk.* **54**, 333.
1925. RAEDER, J. G. *Klin. Monatsbl. f. Augenheilk.* **74**, 424.
1925. NEAME, H. and WAJID ALI KHAN. *Brit. Jl. of Ophthal.* **9**, 618.
1926. JAENSCH, P. A. *Klin. Monatsbl. f. Augenheilk.* **76**, 433.
1926. FRIEDENWALD, J. S. *Contrib. Ophthal. Science*, Jackson vol. 23.
1926. TERRIEN, F. *Arch. d'Ophtal.* **43**, 385.
1926. GÉRARD, G. and DETROY, L. *Clin. Ophtal.* **30**, 22.
1926. —— *Ann. di Ottal.* **54**, 481.
1926. CHANCE, BURTON. *Amer. Jl. of Ophthal.* **9**, 738, 765.
1928. SEDAN, J. *Ann. d'Ocul.* Aug. **165**, 582.
1929. ARCHANGELSKY, W. *Amer. Jl. of Ophthal.* **12**, 787.

MISLEADING SIGNS

1919. HIRSCHBERG, J. *Centralblatt f. p. Augenheilk.* **41**, 240.
1920. COLLINS, E. TREACHER. *Trans. Ophthal. Soc. U.K.* **40**, 161.
1920. NEAME, HUMPHREY. *Ibid.* **40**, 161.
1920. GREEN, J. *Amer. Jl. of Ophthal.* Discussion, **3**, 732.

1920. FRANCIS, L. M. *Amer. Jl. of Ophthal.* 3, 872.
1921. HEYMANS, M. B. *Arch. d'Ophtal.* 38, 479.
1921. DOESSCHATE, G. *Amer. Jl. of Ophthal.* 4, 607.
1921. FUCHS, A. *Zeitschr. f. Augenheilk.* 46, 230.
1922. LEVY, L. *Amer. Jl. of Ophthal.* 5, 24.
1922. REDAELLI, F. *Ophthal. Year Book* (abstract), 18, 509.
1922. VELHAGEN, C. K. *Klin. Monatsbl. f. Augenheilk.* 68, 89.
1922. CRIGLER, L. W. *Arch. of Ophthal.* 51, 400.
1922. v. HIPPEL, E. *Ber. ü. d. Versamml. d. deutsch. ophth. Gesellsch.* Jena.
1922. —— *Klin. Monatsbl. f. Augenheilk.* 68, 395.
1922. DAWSON, H. G. *Brit. Med. Jl.* 757.
1923. HEINE, L. *Arch. f. Ophthal.* 111, 33.
1923. ROWAN, J. *Trans. Ophthal. Soc. U.K.* 43, 378.
1923. RÖNNE, H. *Acta. ophthal.* 1, 268.
1923. GRISCOM, J. M. *Amer. Jl. of Ophthal.* 5, 690.
1923. ROLLET and BUSSY. *Ann. d'Ocul.* 160, 149.
1923. USHER, C. H. *Brit. Jl. of Ophthal.* 7, 10.
1924. MAWAS, M. *Bull. de l'Assoc. franç. pour l'Étude du Cancer*, Dec.
1924. BUTLER, T. H. and ASSINDER, E. W. *Brit. Jl. of Ophthal.* 8, 321.
1924. MICHAEL, D. *Ophthal. Year Book* (abstract), 20, 341.
1924. MARIN AMAT, M. *Ibid.* (abstract), 20, 343.
1924. WEBB-JOHNSON, A. E. and McLEOD, C. E. *Brit. Med. Jl.* 314.
1924–5. COHEN, M. *N.Y. State Jl. of Med.* 24, 707.
1925. MAWAS, M. *Bull. de l'Assoc. franç. pour l'Étude du Cancer*, March.
1925. RÖNNE, H. *Ophthal. Year Book* (abstract), 21, 235.
1925. PETERFI, M. *Zeitschr. f. Augenheilk.* 55, 118.
1925. REESE, W. S. *Amer. Jl. of Ophthal.* 8, 865.
1925. NITSCH, M. *Zeitschr. f. Augenheilk.* 57, 225.
1925. GAMBLE, R. *Amer. Jl. of Ophthal.* 8, 662.
1926. SHOEMAKER, W. J. *Contrib. Ophthal. Science*, Jackson vol. 146.
1926. SEEFELDER, R. *Arch. f. Augenheilk.* 97, 149.
1926. HOLTH, S. *Klin. Monatsbl. f. Augenheilk.* 76, 510.
1926. TERRIEN, F. *Arch. d'Ophtal.* 43, 386.
1926. MERKEL, F. *Arch. f. Augenheilk.* 97, 294.
1926. CHANCE, BURTON. *Amer. Jl. of Ophthal.* 9, 765.
1926. HOWARD, C. N. *Trans. Amer. Acad. Ophthal. Oto-Lar.*
1927. SCHWARTZ, F. O. *Amer. Jl. of Ophthal.* 10, 35.
1927. DOHERTY, W. B. *Ibid.* Jan. 10, 1.
1927. STICHERLING, W. *Roentgen Rays Therapy of Glioma*, Thesis, Freiburg.
1928. CHANCE, BURTON. *Amer. Jl. of Ophthal.* 11, 859.
1928. DOHERTY, W. B. *Trans. Amer. Ophthal. Soc.* 26, 309.
1928. v. HIPPEL, E. *Klin. Monatsbl. f. Augenheilk.* 81, 30.
1929. KOLIOPOULOS. *Ann. d'Ocul.* 166, 206.
1929. JOHNSON, K. B. *Brit. Jl. of Ophthal.* 13, 498.
1929. ELLETT, E. C. *Amer. Jl. of Ophthal.* 12, 681.

1929. Grosz, E. *Arch. f. Augenheilk.* **100-1**, 236.
1930. Moore, R. Foster. *Brit. Jl. of Ophthal.* **14**, 145.
1930. Ellett, E. C. *Amer. Jl. of Ophthal.* **13**, 47.

METASTATIC CARCINOMA OF CHOROID

1923. Maggiore, L. *Rev. gén. d'Ophtal.* **37**, 216.
1923. Usher, C. H. *Brit. Jl. of Ophthal.* **7**, 10.
1924. Adrogué, E. *Ophthal. Year Book* (abstract), **20**, 341.
1925. Knapp, A. *Arch. of Ophthal.* **54**, 389.
1925. Fileti, A. *Ann. di Ottal.* **54**, 596.
1925. Gamble, R. *Amer. Jl. of Ophthal.* **8**, 662.
1926. Usher, C. H. *Brit. Jl. of Ophthal.* **10**, 180.
1926. Clapp, C. A. *Amer. Jl. of Ophthal.* **9**, 513.
1926. Singer, J. *Klin. Monatsbl. f. Augenheilk.* **77**, 181.
1926. Mulock Houwer, A. W. *Ibid.* **77**, 226.
1926. Elschnig, H. H. *Arch. f. Ophthal.* **117**, 316.
1929. Pollakova, J. *Oft. Sbornik*, **3**, 377.
1930. —— *Amer. Jl. of Ophthal.* March, **13**, 267.

GLIOMA

1898. Rockliffe, W. C. *Trans. Ophthal. Soc. U.K.* **18**, 139.
1898. Clarke, E. *Ibid.* **18**, 136.
1907. Stoewer. *Arch. of Ophthal.* **36**, 824.
1909. Paul, Stumpf and Sicherer. *Beitr. zur Geburtsh. und Gynnak.* **13**, 408.
1919. Maghy, C. A. *Brit. Jl. of Ophthal.* **3**, 337.
1920. Fernandez. *Rev. Cub. d'Oftal.* **7**, 30.
1922. Aubineau and Opin. *Arch. d'Ophtal.* **39**, April.
1924. Jacobs. *Jl. Amer. Med. Assoc.* **83**, 164.
1926. v. Leber, Th. *Graefe-Saem. Handbuch*, part 2, **11**, 1453.
1926. Friedenwald, J. S. *Contrib. Ophthal. Science*, Jackson vol. 23.
1926. Sattler, H. *Bosartigen Geschwulste des Auges.*
1926. Gérard, G. and Detroy, L. *Clin. Ophthal.* **30**, 328.
1927. Lachman, G. S. *Amer. Jl. of Ophthal.* March, **10**, 164.
1929. Verhoeff, F. H. *Arch. of Ophthal.* **2**, 643.

CHAPTER V

TREATMENT

PROPHYLACTIC TREATMENT

As retinal detachment appears to be intimately associated with myopic degeneration in middle and advanced life it is wise to emphasise the importance of prophylaxis. Stallard quotes Nordenson's statistics, in which 80 per cent. of a series of 1100 patients with spontaneous detachment of the retina were myopes, and of these 50 per cent. were over fifty years of age. So the main aim of prophylaxis is the prevention of myopia, of its advance, and consequent degeneration. All myopes, preferably all patients, and more particularly all patients of school age, should be instructed in ocular hygiene. The illumination should enable print to be read without effort, and should shine from behind. Print should be clear, properly spaced, and on a matt paper. The book should lie on a sloped desk, or be arranged in some other way that will lead to a minimum of strain on the elevators and depressors of the globe. It should not be closer than 33 cm., so that no undue strain is imposed on the muscles of convergence. This requires adaptation of the chair and table to the size of the patient. Memory work should be encouraged, and the introduction of intervals for ocular rest during the study period should be made. Stallard wisely advocates that progressive myopes should abstain from games that are likely to cause blows, jerks or excessive straining. Bandaging and care are necessary after any severe contusion, especially as detachments can occur some time after the injury. A holiday in the country can be of great value if taken at a suitable time. The following case is no less important because common. A girl aged thirteen years, who was slightly hypermetropic four years before, developed 3 D. of myopia. At each visit the myopia appeared to have increased. She was sent to the country for six months, and encouraged to refrain from near work. Three years later her refraction was the same as it was when she left school for the country. The myopia appeared to be completely arrested.

Grunert's method of treating myopia with pilocarpine is at least worth a trial. He used either drops or ointment. The strength was varied according to the degree of myopia. In myopia up to 6 D. $\frac{1}{5}$ to $\frac{1}{3}$ per cent. was used. In myopia of from 6 to 12 D. $\frac{1}{2}$ per cent. was used, and if the myopia was over 12 D., 1–2 per cent. was usually recommended. The most striking results were in the last group, partly because patients with high myopia are impelled by anxiety to carry out thorough treatment for a sufficiently long period. Of 399 patients with myopia of less than 6 D., 54 per cent. were progressive when not treated with pilocarpine, whereas amongst fifty-three with a corresponding degree of myopia 41·5 per cent. were progressive when treated. Of ninety-nine patients with from 6 to 12 D., 54·5 per cent. advanced when not treated, compared with 8 per cent. of a series of twenty-six who were treated. Of thirty-eight myopes of over 12 D., 91 per cent. advanced without treatment, but only 6·6 per cent. of sixty patients did so when treated with pilocarpine. Pains in the head, "asthenopia dolorosa", can be removed with absolute certainty, according to Grunert. He has given up Fukala's operation (removal of the lens), repeated paracentesis, and subconjunctival injections. Meller (1929), in a recent report of two patients, stated that the intracapsular extraction of lenses in myopia was less dangerous than needling.

The artificial interruption of pregnancy for high-grade myopia is a point of importance at times. Birch-Hirschfeld (1929) considers this indicated if one eye is seriously affected by myopic degeneration and definite changes are present in the other. The wise course to adopt in pregnancy, after re-attachment of a detachment, will depend on the state of the other eye.

CONSERVATIVE MEASURES. Under certain conditions a trial of non-operative treatment is indicated. In all recent traumatic cases, unless a tear is visible, this is wise. The vitreous is often blood-stained, and as it clears a tear may be revealed. If obvious signs of retinitis or choroiditis are present, or if one considers that a certain septic focus may have played some part, one is justified in delaying operation if one thoroughly attempts to eradicate the cause. If a detachment is seen during the first few days, one should reserve operation. If the separation lessens, successful conservative treatment is more probable. If, however, it advances, operation is indicated. Gonin advises operation as soon as possible. It is almost always unwise to wait until the exudate has descended. During its descent it may cause permanent damage to the retina. Whilst waiting, the detachment may become more extensive. Even so, many operators advise delay. Hirschberg advised ten weeks in bed prior to any operation. Fehr, Deutschmann and Uhthoff advise more or less delay and the use of conservative measures but, in the light of Gonin's reports, one must operate early.

REST. This has always been considered to be one of the essentials in treating detachment of the retina. Fortunately improved methods of operative technique have made it unnecessary now to condemn patients to six weeks of immobility on the back, with the head between sandbags. When one remembers the path taken by the fluid, it appears unwise to lay the patient on the back once the fluid has reached the inferior pole of the globe. Unless adhesions have formed around it, the exudate may gravitate to the macular region as one sees a boat-shaped subhyaloid haemorrhage become discoid about the macula when the patient is put on the back. Leber considered rest of little or no avail if the exudate had sunk to the inferior pole of the eye.

It seems to me that once the fluid has been removed by operation, one should use the weight of the vitreous to press the retina against the choroid. So it is important to keep the patient with a detachment of the retina in the inferior pole sitting up in Fowler's position, the end of the bed raised on blocks one foot in height. Similarly the patient who has had a puncture done in the upper pole for a detachment of the retina should, for the first few days, be nursed with the head down. This cannot be done for long, because the patient finds the position too uncomfortable. One has but to observe the sagging down of a persistent hyaloid artery, or the settling down of vitreous opacities, to realise the importance of this point. It is less important probably if a tear is present, and the retina is simply floating in vitreous.

Immobility of the eye is of more importance than immobility of the body. Bandaging of both eyes is essential to gain this. The pressure of this bandage must be sufficient to immobilise and yet not to compress, unless extra pressure is desired, according to the principles to be mentioned later.

Stargardt (1922), besides operation, recommends that attention be given to the best possible lighting of the eye, as an illuminated retina holds more firmly to the choroid than an unilluminated one.

To show the value of rest, Vogt (1928) quotes the following history. A myope (— 2·75 D.S.), aged sixty-five, developed a detachment in his only useful eye. The other had been blind for several years from a similar cause. After fifteen months of treatment including rest, bandaging and saline injections, the condition was unchanged, and a large tear was visible. Rest, however, was continued for a year, and the edges of the tear gradually became re-attached. The vision five years later was 6/4.

Guibert's patient (1924) is of interest. The patient spent three months in bed during an attack of typhoid, and the detachment re-attached completely. (See also Anklesaria, 1929.)

The patient's head must be immobilised in the most suitable position, and any exertion or any tendency to constipation, coughing or sneezing should be checked.

DRUGS. The object of therapeutic measures is to aid the absorption of the inter-retinal fluid. The drugs worth trying are mercury salts, sodium salicylate, iodides and pilocarpine. Kerry (1928, 1929) reports success after the internal use of iodine. Lamb and Ziegler (1921) advocated the use of thyroid (gr. ½ t.d.s.) believing that it increased the flow of aqueous. It certainly lessens the tendency to haemorrhage in myxoedema, and the presence of this as a cause of subretinal haemorrhage is worth remembering. The application of X-rays has been reported of value in aiding resorption of fluid, and so playing a part in the cure of retinal detachment (Vigano, 1921). The value of venesection or the application of leeches has been stressed by Aschner (1929), Jablonski (1929) and Hamburger (1928).

COMPRESSION BANDAGE. This has long been recommended as an aid in the treatment of detachment of the retina. A brief consideration of its effects shows that it is important to consider the degree of compression desirable, and that it is unwise to use it in all cases. Samelsohn (1875) was the first to emphasise the value of compression. He, however, twelve years later (1887), was forced to admit that lasting and complete cures were very rare. Wessely (1905) reported an excellent result. The patient was a high myope with a detachment of the whole of the retina except the inferior nasal quadrant. Twice after ceasing treatment the detachment recurred, but finally complete and apparently permanent re-attachment ensued.

What is the effect on the eye of externally applied pressure? E. E. Henderson and Starling showed that the escape of fluid was increased from animals' eyes if intra-ocular pressure was raised to 50–60 mm. Hg. Ballantyne showed a fall of tension if the tonometer was left on an eye for a few seconds. Hine has shown that the intra-ocular pressure varies with the amount of pressure applied by a pressure bandage, and that in the majority of eyes, tension returns to normal in about one and a half hours. Schmelzer (1929) has noticed only a very slight reduction of tension, when the 10 or 15 grm. weight of a tonometer is left on a glaucomatous eye. So we can agree with Parsons when he says that prolonged pressure, externally applied, gradually squeezes fluid out from the eye. This fluid includes blood from the choroid. Magitot and Bailliart (1922) consider that the main effect is the emptying of the choroidal system and that normal tension returns as, little by little, the vessels refill, and the pressure again becomes normal. "On removing the external pressure the tension remains low until increased secretion produces compensation—a comparatively slow process." It is well to remember here the extreme vascularity of the choroid, and that its innermost tissue is an elastic membrane—lamina vitrea or membrane of Bruch. This permits of great variation in the capacity of the choroid.

It appears that pressure on a normal eye will tend to reduce the volume of the whole eye and the colloidal vitreous. If a detachment of the retina is present, the pressure can act favourably only if the volume-retaining tendency of the vitreous is at least as great as the volume-retaining tendency of the subretinal space and there is a pressure of the vitreous against the retina. If the vitreous is very fluid, and it usually is, if there is a retinal tear, pressure bandages would appear to be useless.

In applying the bandage, one must consider the position of the eye in the socket, and its relation to the orbital margin. This as a rule prevents the application of a constant pressure. To obviate this, Comberg has attempted to regulate the pressure manometrically and to vary it as required. One must guard against too marked a fall in tension after removing the bandage, by applying only moderate pressure, and that for not more than half an hour at a time. There can be no value in this method once the intra-ocular pressure falls below that of subretinal space. Wessely (1922) demonstrated, experimentally on animals, that no beneficial effect followed such bandaging. Mendoza (1920) makes a plaster mould of the eye and orbital ridges for each patient and uses this in bandaging. Gonin (1921) objects to the compression bandage, applied according to Samelsohn, because it is apt to produce superficial keratitis and cyclitis, and because it is rarely tolerated. He considers that a bandage should be immobilising, but not compressive. Leber reported the development of acute hypotony and a "peculiar form of iridocyclitis" after too long or too firm an application of a compression bandage. It appears most likely that these results are due to absorption of the inter-retinal fluid by the choroidal vessels.

DIET. It may be wise to restrict the intake of fluids. Excessive drinking of water is contra-indicated. The diet should be well balanced and so constituted that any tendency to constipation and the associated straining will be lessened. The tendency to oedema in patients with a defective and a deficient protein intake during the war suggests the need to watch for this in poverty-stricken patients. Joslin points out that "a diet rich in carbohydrate brings about an increase in weight, whereas a diet of exactly the same number of calories, though chiefly made up of fat, lowers the weight". These changes are due simply to the retention of water by the tissues in the one case, and to its loss in the other. This suggests a possible advantage in increasing the proportion of fat to carbohydrate. Marx (1922) advocates the use of a salt-free diet. He supports this by theoretical and experimental data. Hertel has proved that intra-ocular pressure increased in a rabbit's eye when hypotonic saline was infused. Believing that the ciliary body secretes fluid, Marx considers that if there is no salt intake, the amount of fluid is increased. The consequent increase in the bulk of the vitreous will force the retina against the choroid. Marx has adopted this diet during eleven years, and reports ten cures. Three of these were old cases. In all, the improvement was gradual and no other method was adopted. He considers that the outlook is not so good in nephritis, because of the tendency to oedema, due to the retention of sodium chloride. Noiszewski (1923) has used chlorine-free diet ever since he found that many patients with retinal detachment showed a marked reduction in the total chlorides in the urine. He reported two complete cures. In one case the condition was bilateral and it had resisted all other methods of treatment. The other patient was a boy who was cured after two months of this diet. Stargardt (1922) recommended the use of calcium chloride. Intravenous calcium chloride at first greatly increases the production of ocular fluid, and then causes a prolonged reduction. Calcium salts appear to have the power of decreasing the permeability of vessels and of contracting the smaller ones (Rochat and Steijn, 1924; Tristaino, 1922). Therefore they may play a part in lessening the tendency to effusion from a congested choroid.

OPERATIVE TREATMENT

The number and diversity of the operative measures used for treating detachments of the retina suggest their inefficacy. A study of the results certainly confirms this idea. The operations vary according to the operator's own conception of the mechanism which produced the separation. One objective common to most operations has been the removal of the inter-retinal fluid. Other additional objectives have been sought by different men in various ways. These aims can be summarised as follows:

To excite the formation of adhesions.

To divide the vitreous strands.

To reduce the capacity of the globe.

To provide permanent drainage.

To raise the tension or to increase the bulk of the vitreous.

And to close the tear or retinal aperture.

THE FORMATION OF ADHESIONS. The removal of the fluid was considered essential by all those who postulated a serous choroiditis as the initial lesion. If the fluid is a product of inflammation, it may have properties which will affect the vitality of the retina. This "exudation" theory originated various measures which were intended to increase the absorptive power of the body. These are purgation, sweating by the injection of pilocarpine and by hot air baths, the administration of iodides and salicylates, subconjunctival injections and others.

The operative measures adopted to drain the subretinal fluid include simple aspiration, scleral cauterisation with or without retinal puncture, trephining and other endeavours to maintain permanent drainage by the insertion of gold wire or horsehair. Just as the puncture appears to start resorption in pleurisy, so a puncture may act when some of the fluid is removed from under the retina (Elschnig).

Meyer Wiener (1924), in an interesting paper, states that in 1805 James Ware advocated scleral puncture for the relief of detachment of the retina. Hancock in 1860 made a sclerotomy with a knife or a needle, and then cut through the ciliary muscle. Von Graefe (1863) reported a series of fifty cases in which he punctured not only the sclera, but also the retina. His aim was to drain the subretinal fluid into the vitreous. Eighteen months after the operation only four cases showed improvement. At first the sclera only was punctured but von Graefe, seeing the futility of this, and realising that detachment with spontaneous tear showed a slight but definite tendency to heal, suggested retinal puncture. The results from this method were not encouraging. De Wecker and Abadie (1881–2) were amongst the first to use the thermo-cautery in the treatment of detachment of the retina but their results were not satisfactory. Years later this method was made popular by the results of H. Dor (1895–1907). He combined scleral cauterisation with strong saline injections, occasional bleedings, and sweating. Though his early results were promising—nine cures amongst fifteen patients—later (1907), only 30 per cent. were considered cured. He admitted, however, that mostly early cases were treated. Here lies the important pitfall in considering the percentage of cures. Some writers have included only early cases, some even puerperal cases, and their results are not comparable with those who treated all cases except those associated with pregnancy. Many cases if watched longer would be found to be very transient cures. This is emphasised by the report of L. Dor (1907). He reported twenty-five patients he had treated. He combined scleral-puncture with his father's method of treatment in ten of these. 48 per cent. were considered immediate cures, but later only 8 per cent. were found to be permanent. Finally, 56 per cent. were classed as definite failures, and of these a very high percentage developed irido-cyclitis (nine out of fourteen cases) and required enucleation. As a result of his experience and of the experiments of others he was satisfied that the cauterisation of the sclera alone was sufficient to excite an "adhesive inflammation". It was doubtful whether this would be sufficient to cause the resorption of the fluid, or whether this should be drained off. Ever since the experiments of Scheffels (1894) and Wernicke (1906) it had been known that after the scleral cauterisation of a rabbit's eye, a detachment

would form which would disappear in a few weeks, leaving
the three tunics of the eye adherent, and complete atrophy
of the retina and choroid at the site of cauterisation. The
secondary detachment in the lower pole would remain unchanged for much longer, because no absorptive or adhesive
reaction had been initiated there. Possibly Dor's percentage
of irido-cyclitis after cauterisation was high because no
attempt was made to remove the inter-retinal fluid, which
would be greatly increased by the cauterisation. This reaction appears to be greatest in those cases which are probably
due to choroiditis, as for example, those that are associated
with episcleritis or other ocular or general infections. Therefore if one decides to cauterise the sclera, it is essential also
to drain off the fluid. As the human sclera is much thicker
than the rabbit's, and as the retina when detached may be a
considerable distance from the site of scleral cauterisation, it
may remain unaffected by this operation unless it too is perforated. Handmann (1923) examined an eye that had been
cauterised, and found well-established adhesions between
the sclera and the choroid, but the retina was not adherent.
Inter-retinal fluid still existed. These considerations and experimental works convinced operators, especially Sourdille
and others of the French school, that the main difficulties in
re-applying and re-attaching the retina in its former position
were due not only to the presence of the fluid but also to the
retraction of the retina. They considered that even though it
contains no elastic tissue, the muscular coat of the retinal
vessels is sufficient to make it retract, once it is separated from
the choroid. The tendency of this elastic coat is to draw the
retina in the direction of the chord of the arc which the
vessels assumed before separation occurred. To overcome
this difficulty, retinal perforation with a knife or cautery was
added to the multiple punctures of the outer coats of the eyeball which had been in vogue for a time (Sourdille, 1923,
1929). This additional measure enabled the retina to expand
again into its former position and it provided a permanent
drain for the subretinal fluid. Sourdille plunged a Graefe
knife 10–12 mm. into the eye at three or four points opposite
the detachment. The inter-retinal fluid was allowed to escape

by rotating the knife through ninety degrees before with-drawing it. Sourdille then injected mercury cyanide (1–1000) into the oedematous conjunctiva. During the patient's stay of three weeks in hospital, 6 per cent. saline was injected at weekly intervals. Later he modified his procedure by again puncturing the eye, using fine electric needles, four weeks after the first operation. By these means he endeavoured to produce adhesions. Sourdille considered that it took two months at least for firm adhesions to form. His patients were warned against stooping and straining. Near work was allowed in very gradually increasing amounts. As relapses occurred in two patients after long train journeys, these were forbidden. He was in favour of early operation, considering three months to be the limit after which complete recovery was most unlikely. In treating sixteen recent detachments, he reported nine lasting cures. These were followed for periods of from six months to two years. His standard of vision was ability to read with ease. Of eighteen patients with detachments of from four to thirteen months' duration at least, he claimed 50 per cent. lasting improvement. Gallois (1926) claimed two cures out of six detachments, when using Sourdille's methods. Walker (1925) had one excellent result, after making five punctures through sclera and retina 10 mm. posterior to the lower border of the cornea with a discission needle. The needle was turned at right angles at the last puncture to allow the fluid to escape. More recently this method (i.e. cauterisation) has been combined with excision of a small part of the sclera (Birch-Hirschfeld). Thiel (1928) reports sixty-seven patients treated at the Berlin Clinic during the two and a half years ending July 1928. Neither medical treatment (eighteen patients), nor treatment by puncture alone (twenty patients), showed permanent success. Cauterisation was used in twenty-nine patients. Five were completely cured, though the return of full vision was the exception. Sometimes Stargardt's method of puncturing with the cautery was used; at other times Löhlein's method was adopted (superficial cauterisation followed by puncture with a knife). Many methods to promote adhesions have been suggested. Electrolysis of the inter-retinal fluid was used by many operators thirty-five years ago (Terson, 1895; and Montgomery, 1896; Clavelier and Maravel, 1895; Snell, 1896; Lagrange, 1897; Clavelier, 1897; Maravel, 1901). Their results were not encouraging. Stallard (1930) recently was able to collect seven patients treated in this way, of whom 10 per cent. were cured. An equal percentage were considered to be improved. Other methods in vogue for a time were the injection of irritating fluids under the detachment, the puncture of the retina in various ways, and the making of large equatorial incisions in the retina (Sachs). Little if any success is reported as the result of these measures. They may produce fine scarring, but once the delicate connections between the rods and cones and the pigment epithelium are atrophic, it is a poor substitute for the normal attachments. Special mention must be made of the courageous attempts made by Galezowski (1890), Martin and Evers, who sutured the choroid to the retina with catgut, horsehair, and silk.

SUBCONJUNCTIVAL INJECTIONS. Subconjunctival injections of hypertonic saline have been widely used. They were first used by Mellinger (1896). He used from 4 to 10 per cent. saline and gave at least ten injections. He obtained two cures amongst fifteen patients. Favourable results have been reported after the use of varying strengths. Ramsay (1906) reported 12 per cent. marked improvements (probable cures) and 18 per cent. moderate improvements in the treatment of fifty patients. Occasionally he combined puncture with his routine injection (3 per cent. saline with ½ per cent. oxycyanide of mercury). H. Dor (1896) used stronger and even 35 per cent. saline, and advised injections under Tenon's capsule. Foster Moore (1921) gave nine injections under Tenon's capsule of 15 minims every third day. He used 5 per cent. sodium chloride and 5 per cent. sodium citrate with 4 per cent. novocaine alternately. During the years 1923 and 1927, twelve patients were treated by this method. Only one showed any improvement. In one the vitreous opacities increased, and in another a cataract developed (Stallard, 1930). Parsons recommended the use of 10 per cent. saline. Tristaino (1922) considered that by combining sodium chloride with dionine he obtained better results, whilst de Wecker used gelatin and normal saline. Herkel (1922) and Marquez (1915) claim improvement and cure from the use of sodium chloride alone. With a view to promoting the formation of adhesions, mercury oxycyanide (1–3 minims of from 1–1000 to 1–4000) or dionine from ½ per cent. to 5 per cent. have been given. Darier (1920) treated sixty patients mainly by this method. Of these ten were cured and twenty improved. If he considered that the detachment was due to choroiditis, intravenous injections of salicylarsenate of mercury, and subconjunctival injections of 2 per cent. guaiacol were given. Of forty-three patients, seven were reported cured, and eleven improved. Terrien (1922) advised the use of 1–2 c.c. of 3 or 4 per cent. saline every fourth or sixth day. The addition of acoin or novocain renders the injection practically painless.

One object of these injections has been the drainage of the inter-retinal fluid by osmosis. As Stallard has pointed out, the subretinal fluid is mainly colloidal in nature, and the injected solution is a crystalloid solution. The passage of the large colloid molecules through the choroid and sclera, acting as dialysing membrane, would occur with great difficulty, if at all. If the inter-retinal fluid was drained in this way, would not the tissue fluid or aqueous refill the space? If benefit results from this method, it is by the formation of adhesions after the sclera and choroid have been punctured and the fluid drained off.

THE DIVISION OF VITREOUS STRANDS. If the theory of exudation had little anatomical basis, the reverse held for the next theory which was productive of operative measures. The theory of traction was originated and developed by such eminent histologists as Leber and his school, Müller, de Wecker, and Nordenson. Sourdille considered that nothing but failure could attend measures based on a theory which was the product of laboratory investigations of old detached retinae. The results certainly did not bear out the claims of the ardent exponents of this theory. Deutschmann claimed 20 per cent. cures, but almost universal failure followed the adoption of his method. It consisted in cutting the fibrous strands that existed in the vitreous, and in separating the adhesions between this structure and the retina. Later, after dividing these fine strands, he advocated and practised the injection of rabbits' vitreous. The attempt to sever any fibrous band may increase the detachment by pulling the retina. He later (1895) advocated the making of several incisions in the region of the ora serrata. The object was to reduce the tension on the retina which he considered hindered re-attachment. As Lister says, a single definite band, as cause, is a great rarity. Von Hippel's case is as brilliant as it is unique. He divided a vitreous strand, and the retina re-attached and useful vision returned. So this method is further limited by the great infrequency of the condition in which it is indicated. Finally Deutschmann (1930) through holding that a tear is nature's method of relieving an overstretched retina, and not the condition *sine qua non* for detachment, believes that Gonin's method of treatment is the best for recent detachments.

THE REDUCTION OF OCULAR CAPACITY. When Müller failed to repeat successfully Deutschmann's operation, he advocated a new measure based on the same theory. Finding it impossible to bring the retina into contact with the choroid by division of the vitreous strands, he attempted to bring the choroid in towards the displaced retina by removing a portion of the sclera. The outer half of the sclera is removed over an area of 20 × 10 mm. At the posterior boundary, the sclera is divided completely, and the choroid separated from it. The anterior thinned area of sclera is then inserted posteriorly between choroid and sclera, and the edges of the scleral wound joined by suturing. The technique is difficult, and the risk of haemorrhage and vitreous loss considerable. By so reducing the volume of the eyeball, he hoped to establish adhesions between the two retinal layers, and so restore the function of the rods and cones. Though some success attended this method, it is practically never adopted now. Török stated in 1917 that in the previous twenty-five years only about fifty operations had been reported. He had performed it on twenty-one patients, but could claim no permanent cures. Koch (1927) used this method for eighteen patients, and obtained one complete and permanent cure, and improvement in six others.

THE PROVISION OF PERMANENT DRAINAGE. All this time Gonin was emphasising the idea that the retinal tear was the essential feature. However, progress was slow, and the methods advocated increased in diversity. Trephining the eye was neglected after de Wecker in 1872, and Argyll Robertson in 1876 reported their results. When Elliot modified and perfected the excellent operation which bears his name, it was soon considered a possible means of establishing permanent drainage for the inter-retinal fluid. It was thought that if the sclera was trephined over the site of detachment, it would give permanent drainage to the inter-retinal space, and so prevent the further collection of fluid. Hessberg (1924), Lambert (1923), and many others claim little or no success from this method, while MacCallan (1926) and Lawson considered it of value. Ohm (1919) reported two cures in a series of seven patients whom he trephined. Parker (1915) reported fifteen trephines, after which he could only claim four improvements. Thomson and Curtin (1916) recommended that ten days after trephining the inter-retinal fluid should be aspirated. They repeated this, if necessary, as long as the scleral opening remained patent. Two of three patients so treated were improved. Later (1920) they trephined, and aspirated at the same time. They insisted on the complete removal of all the fluid. Of seventy-five patients operated on, seven were successful. Chipman (1921) reported one cure and one improvement when he trephined and aspirated according to the method suggested by Thomson. Damel (1921) also reported a cure. Unfortunately the trephine hole does not remain open for long, for fibrous tissue soon closes it, and drainage then ceases. Years before, Galezowski (1890) attempted to establish a permanent drain by passing a fine gold wire through and through the conjunctiva, sclera and choroid. This he tied over the conjunctiva, but infection always led to the loss of the eye. Meyer Wiener (1924) to overcome this difficulty makes two openings 1 mm. apart, and inserts a strand of horsehair in one opening. He endeavoured to pass it between the retina and the choroid through the other opening. A full curved needle was used and the horsehair was cut off leaving 1·5 mm. projecting from each trephine opening. Wiener considered that the reduction in tension was one danger following this procedure. He reported two patients with complete re-attachment, out of seven operated on.

Choriodo-dialysis and Holth's pre-equatorial sclerectomy were recommended with a similar end in view. Meller (1923) describes the former operation. He opens the sclera, and with a spatula separates it from the choroid. Then a perforation is made in the choroid, through which the subretinal fluid will escape. It is hoped that it will then be absorbed, and that haemorrhage will lead to the adhesion of the choroid and retina. Sloan (1926) reported two detachments which he had cured by this method. Holth recommends that a 2·5 mm. disc of the sclera be removed by trephining anterior to the equator, and between the inferior and external recti muscles. The supra-choroidal space then communicates with the space within Tenon's capsule. It is hoped that before the opening closes the drainage of the intra-ocular fluid through the choroid will be so increased that the subretinal fluid will be absorbed. Groenholm (1921) reported thirty-six eyes on which he had performed this operation. He claimed 10 per cent. cures. In a considerable number the condition appeared worse. La Ferla reported his experiences with this method.

THE RAISING OF THE INTRA-OCULAR TENSION. A series of operations has been adopted with a view to raising the intra-ocular tension, and so exerting pressure on the retina when it is reapplied. Of those, Lagrange's operation—*colmatage*—is worthy of mention. It was recommended in 1912 by Lagrange. Since then van Heuven (1926), Csapody (1928), Pesme (1921), Delorme (1923), Birch-Hirschfeld (1928), von Rotth (1929), Foder (1929), have used it with success. Lagrange advised the dissection of a conjunctival flap, posteriorly from the limbus, and the making of a triple row of scleral cautery punctures round the limbus. He and Csapody considered that the rise in tension, which followed this measure, was due to the constriction by a cicatricial ring of Schlemm's canal. Van Heuven, when discussing this operation, stated that he considered the increased tension was due to the increase in the albumen content of the aqueous, and the hyperaemia produced which lasts from ten to twenty days. Experimentally he found that the tension in rabbits remained raised for six months sometimes. He does not expect good results in old cases, or in very myopic or aphakic eyes. Van Heuven reported six recent detachments which were definitely improved. The best result was in a very recent traumatic case. He operated on the upper half of the eyeball first, and five days later on the lower. Delorme treated a series of thirty detachments; twenty-two of these he considered due to myopia, and of these raised tension was produced in eighteen, with twelve complete re-attachments and full visual fields in nine. Four were considered due to serous exudation, and of these two developed full fields. He stripped the conjunctiva towards the limbus and cauterised the episcleral tissues. He combined it with four subconjunctival injections of 10 per cent. saline at intervals of five days after the operations. He injected between the muscles behind the equator. Pesme reported fifteen cures in a series of twenty-seven detachments. These cases were not followed for long. Deutschmann claimed that any benefit resulting from this operation was due to the puncture. The raised tension could only cure, if low tension was the cause, and this he disbelieves. Kümmell welcomed this operation because he considered hypotony to be the most important fundamental sign. Löwenstein (1923) recommended this method. Wieden (1921) and del Castillo (1923) were not successful with this operation.

Bettremieux (1928–9) recommends an operation which probably acts in a similar way to "colmatage", though he considers that by opening up the venous spaces round the cornea, the intra-ocular circulation and nutrition are improved. He states that "non-perforating pericorneal sclerectomy" should be the first step in treating detachment. He considers the operation so efficacious if the detachment is due to choroiditic effusion, that if it were performed for choroiditis, it would prevent the development of a detachment. A preliminary rise in tension follows. It is difficult to see why the author also recommends this measure in "haemorrhagic glaucoma". He dissects up the conjunctiva from the limbus and leaves

bare an area 15-18 mm. wide. He then removes a strip
2 × 18 mm. of superficial tissue round the limbus and replaces the conjunctival flap. New anastomoses form and so
improve the nutrition of the choroid, and he claims also that
of the retina. This operation can be repeated at other points
round the limbus (Vitou, 1925). Van Heuven has shown that
even the loosening of the conjunctiva of a rabbit is sufficient
to raise the ocular tension. Probably any benefit from this
operation is due to this effect. Cauterisation probably is
beneficial, apart from the removal of the fluid, because of
hyperaemia induced in the choroid. Subconjunctival injections may be of value for the same reason. Stargardt believes in immediate operation, and the application of a hot,
but not a red-hot, cautery to the choroid which has been exposed by dissecting off the sclera. He administers calcium
chloride, and does not exclude light from the eye, considering
that the illuminated retina is more firmly adherent to the
choroid than when light is excluded.

With a view to increasing the bulk of the contents of the
vitreous chamber, and so pressing the retina against the
choroid, the intra-ocular injection of various substances has
been tried. Some used cerebro-spinal fluid. Birch-Hirschfeld, Wood (1920), and others used the inter-retinal fluid
itself, and others used saline and various other solutions. The
originators of these methods considered that the loss in
volume of the vitreous was probably the main exciting cause
and certainly a hindrance to recovery. However, the effect
of these measures is very transient, and they are poor sub-
stitutes for normal vitreous. Carbone (1924) advocated the
subconjunctival injection of hygrometric fluid and the injection of substances into the anterior chamber which would
obstruct the exit of ocular fluid, viz. bovine vitreous, 0·5-1 per
cent. gelatine or NaCl 1 per cent. in glycerine. Proksch
(1926) injected paraffin and gelatine into the vitreous. Nakashima's (1926) experiments with rabbits, into the vitreous of
which protein bodies and grape sugar were injected, proved
to be risky and of little benefit.

A measure of success attended the injection of air, and for
that reason fuller reference will be made to it. After dissecting

off a conjunctival flap over the area of detachment, one divides Tenon's capsule and retracts it with sutures. Then one bares the sclera in another position, and inserts a fine needle attached to a syringe full of air. This is handed to an assistant who is instructed to watch the tip of the needle, making sure that it does not touch the lens. Then, with a dull red cautery, one slowly burns a hole through the sclera and choroid. This may be done in one or two sites if little fluid flows out. Then taking the syringe, one injects air. The air can be seen to bubble into the vitreous. Then with great care, while pressing back the sclera round it with forceps, one withdraws the needle. Both conjunctival wounds are gently closed with sutures. This method was described by Rohmer (1912). Jeandelize and Baudot (1926) made a series of punctures with a cataract knife, injected 1 c.c. of sterilised air at the edge of the detachment, and then injected a solution containing the oxycyanide of mercury under the conjunctiva. I have operated on only two recent detachments by the former method. Four old ones were not improved. One man, aged seventy, was seen with a superior detachment in his only eye. The other eye had been blind for more than twenty years. It was cataractous, degenerate, and had no perception of light. The eye was punctured by a cautery, air was injected as described above, and the retina was reapplied and remained so for two months. Then one day, after a longer walk than usual, the retina began to separate again. The eye was again cauterised, without further injections of air, but the retina did not completely return into position. One noted after the second operation what others have reported, namely, the development of a transient detachment on the side of the eye opposite the site of cauterisation. Soon afterwards, however, this patient succumbed to an attack of pneumonia, which followed the development of pyelitis and scattered areas of phlebitis. This history demonstrates the advisability of having the co-operation of a physician whenever one confines an elderly patient to bed. The second patient with a recent detachment was a woman aged thirty-seven, who for three and a half months had had the lower half of the retina detached. After a cautery puncture and the injection of air into the vitreous, the retina returned to its former position. As the detachment had been in the lower pole of the eye, the patient was nursed in Fowler's position. When examined last, twenty months after the operation, the retina was still in perfect position.

The ability of the vitreous to swell under certain conditions may lead to some method whereby the retina is pressed back in its original position. Duke-Elder suggests the forcing in of hydrogen ions as a possible means of increasing the turgescence of the vitreous.

THE CLOSING OF THE RETINAL TEAR: GONIN'S TREATMENT. In 1925, Gonin stated that as a result of thermocauterisation he had more cures in three or four years than in the previous twenty-five years. From this method, his new operation developed.

Before describing this great advance in the treatment of an otherwise intractable condition, it is wise to summarise Gonin's views. In 1921 he stated that the best results were obtained by a scleral cautery-puncture. Lasting results, however, were rarely found. It was a last hope, and it was contraindicated if the other eye was blind. In 1920, Jocqs stated that Gonin's views could lead only to therapeutic nihilism. Compare this pessimism with the results to be described shortly.

Gonin (1928 b) states that "spontaneous" retinal detachments are due to the tearing of the retinal tissue by a dragging of the vitreous. He considers that tears are due to localised adhesions between the vitreous and the retina. These adhesions follow an attack of chorio-retinitis which is so common in the equatorial region, and they may be in existence for a long time before a tear develops. If, in addition, there exists a degenerate vitreous, and this is almost the rule in myopia and is frequent in senility, then a varying quantity of a non-albuminous watery fluid replaces part of the vitreous. This lessens the normal support given to the retina and enables any strands, which may exist in the vitreous, to drag on the retina during an ocular movement or bodily effort. As a result a retinal tear results, and if it occurs in a degenerate area extra tears may soon form in that vicinity. The conditions which are essential, according to Gonin, are vitreous liquefaction, adhesions between the vitreous and the retina, and a movement of the vitreous sufficient to exert strain on the more or less degenerate retina and produce a tear. Gonin considers that retinal tears are constant, and can be found in all idiopathic and all traumatic detachments. Vogt found them in twenty-three out of twenty-five relatively recent spontaneous detachments. Gonin states that in 83 per cent. of cases they are situated in the periphery, and that if one can induce choroido-retinal adhesions which close the tear, one will obtain a complete and lasting cure in from ten to fifteen days. He claims that one can arrest an old detachment, but that it is difficult to get perfect re-application. If cures are not obtained it is because either the rent has not been closed or because other tears exist. In one out of ten patients, a series of holes can be found. Multiple tears may develop even during the treatment, if the resistance of the retina is low. Gonin has said, "When the ruptures are too big or too numerous, or when the media are not transparent, one cannot hope for a radical cure". If the detachment is so old that the retina is atrophic, it may not be possible to close the hole. He considers that those who claim that tears are of only secondary importance, and that those who state that the presence of a tear makes the outlook hopeless (Lister, 1924; Holth) are equally wrong. A tear is the cause of many detachments and its closing provides a means of cure. He states that treatment should be adopted as soon as possible, certainly within the first few weeks of the development of the lesion. It appears that Gonin more recently has considered that the ideal time for operation is between the tenth and the twenty-first day.

THE RECOGNITION OF A TEAR. The *first essential* is to find the tear. Great emphasis is laid by visitors to Gonin's clinic, on the painstaking search of the fundus. Occasionally it may be wise to seat the patient on a high chair, so that one may explore the upper periphery. As a rule it is easier to search the periphery of the fundus if the patient is in the horizontal position. Full dilatation of the pupil is desirable. Sometimes euphthalmine gives the best results. The finding of a tear is very difficult if the pupil is resistant to the influence of mydriatics and if the patient finds it difficult to rotate his eye fully. The indirect method of ophthalmoscopy is the best method for searching the periphery of the fundus. This method, because of the prismatic effect due to the spherical lens, gives a wider field than either the direct method or the binocular method of Gullstrand. Vogt uses a lens of $5-5\frac{1}{2}$ cm. diameter, and about 13 D. Pressure on the globe, according to Trantas, may help. Repeated examinations may be necessary, as the tear may be obscured by a retinal fold for a time. It may be revealed only after the patient has been recumbent for several days, or has had certain conservative treatment. It may be very small and simulate a haemorrhage. The retina may be reapplied in part, and the tear lying in this area may be some distance from the remaining detachment. A tear of the upper retina may be associated with an inferior detachment, if the initial detachment has begun to re-attach, and the fluid has yielded to the force of gravity. Therefore one should examine most thoroughly the whole of the fundus, and particularly the area of the fundus which corresponds with the initial field loss, as described by the patient. At times it is not until the inter-retinal fluid has been drawn off by a hypodermic syringe that the tear is revealed. By red-free light, the choroid will appear black, and in marked contrast to the free edge of the tear, which will appear completely opaque.

As already stated, Vogt (1930) does not consider that holes and rents have a similar origin. He considers a horseshoe-shaped hole is intermediate between the two. Generally apertures are more easily detected in moderately than in excessively or deficiently pigmented eyes. They are chiefly found in a zone which is from three to five disc diameters from the ora serrata. Even the smallest hole is of importance. Vogt (1930) has described a detachment which showed a hole only a quarter of a disc diameter (D.D.) in width, the closing of which led to re-attachment. The slowness of onset of this detachment was supposed to be due to the smallness of the hole.

Retinal haemorrhages and choroidal vessels may simulate a tear very closely. The former are found at times on the surface of a detachment. They are a darker red than a tear, and being superficial, are usually flame-shaped and pointed. They do not show the white edge, the parallax or the underlying exposed choroidal vessels which a tear usually does. When a wide choroidal vessel is visible for only a short distance it may resemble a retinal hole. Small atrophic areas in the choroid are usually surrounded by pigment, and as the pigment epithelium has atrophied, they show a paler base than a hole does. Greater difficulty may be found in distinguishing the spaces in cystoid degeneration from actual holes. Vogt emphasises the value of the impression that one gets of the hole being in front of the cyst, that is, on a more anterior plane. It certainly appears to be more prominent. The usual signs of myopic degeneration are frequently found. If the detached retina has become white or greyish, the contrast with the hole is more marked, and it is easier to find.

Vogt describes the occasional appearance of delicate white lines which run approximately parallel to the equator. They are ramified at times, and may appear like moss, or a series of nets. He considers that some of these lines are probably degenerate vessels. The fine branches leaving the main or parent stem do so at right angles. These lines enclose red "obviously thin-partitioned" spaces which are probably cystoid changes. Occasionally one or more of these areas appears as a hole or rent.

THE LOCALISATION OF A TEAR. The *second essential* is to localise the tear. This is often very difficult. Igersheimer, who worked with Gonin for a time, mentions the following pitfalls. Firstly, the possibility of locating the tear incorrectly. Secondly, one may locate it accurately, but not reach it easily with the cautery. Thirdly, it may be too big to close. Fourthly, one or more tears may exist, or arise after treatment. Gonin has found a type of retina which continues to tear after the closing of the first hole. He refers to three such detachments in his series for 1927. Occasionally the retinal folds have become too firm to permit reapplication.

There are several methods of localisation described. Gonin's method will be briefly described first. He says that the only practical means is by the ophthalmoscope, and that the position of the tear can only be determined approximately. Error may be due either to optical fore-shortening when a tear is on the summit of a detached retina, or to the difficulty of knowing exactly where such a hole will actually lie on the choroid when the retina is reapplied. Two relationships of each tear must be noted; *firstly*, the meridian, that is, the sector in which the tear is situated; *secondly*, the parallel circle or the degree of latitude, that is, the distance of the tear from the ora serrata. The determination of the meridian is the simpler. Though Vogt at first calculated the distance of the tear from the disc or the macula, he now adopts Gonin's plan and estimates its distance from the ora serrata. As the eye may rotate during operation (Vogt, 1929 *a*), it is not sufficient to ascertain and refer to the site as if the cornea represented a clock-face. Holocaine anaesthesia of the cornea is desirable, and full dilatation of the pupil is essential. Gonin marks the corneal edge at the two ends of the meridian with an aniline dye. This is quite simple to do if the tear is visible by direct ophthalmoscopy, but more difficult if one can see the tear only by indirect ophthalmoscopy. Rubbrecht (1929), who uses the direct method of ophthalmoscopy, states that when one sees the tear, one moves one's eye and the ophthalmoscope in the direction of the tear until its posterior extremity is just visible, and marks with Indian ink the limbus in line with this. Then one moves in the opposite direction until its anterior limit is just within view, and one marks the opposite part of the limbus in line with this. These points give one the meridian of longitude in which the tear is.

In ascertaining both the degree of latitude and the meridian, it is necessary that the heads of the observer and of the patient should be, as far as possible, on the same level. The correct meridian will be that which enables the heads to be on the same level, when the tear is in the centre of the ophthalmoscopic lens, and this lens is parallel to the iris. If the tear is seen through the edge of the lens, the meridian is not the correct one. When one sees the tear in the centre of the field of observation an assistant works the points where the meridian crosses the limbus. A scratch with a needle dipped in fluorescein suffices. Later Indian ink can be used as a more permanent indicator.

To determine the parallel circle or the degree of latitude, one calculates the number of disc diameters (D.D.) which separate the tear from the ora serrata. As most tears are pre-equatorial, this is simpler than a calculation of the distance from the macula. Gonin considers that the weaker refraction in the periphery and the somewhat oblique direction of vision do not seriously affect the calculation in disc diameters. One error tends to lessen the other. Every apparent D.D. is approximately 1·5 mm. Unfortunately the ora serrata is not visible in every eye, and its distance from the limbus is variable. When invisible one takes the extreme limit that one can see with the ophthalmoscope through a fully dilated pupil. On an average, the distance of the ora serrata from the limbus is 8 mm. In hypermetropia it may be less than 7 mm., and in myopia more than 9. If astigmatism is present, the difference in the two meridians may be 1 or 2 mm. By adding the distance, in millimetres, of the tear from the ora serrata to the distance of the ora serrata from the limbus, 8 mm., one can relate the tear to the limbus. Further measurements of value are: centre of cornea to limbus 5–6 mm., ora serrata to equator 6–7 mm., equator to macula 18–20 mm.

If a tear exists at the ora serrata, it may be localised fairly accurately 8 mm. from the limbus. According to the breadth of the tear (1 or more D.D.), 3 or 4 mm. must be added to 8 mm., and the puncture made at a point 11 or 12 mm. from the limbus. If the tear is found to be 2 D.D. from the ora serrata, one adds $8 + 3 \times 2$, and punctures the sclera 14 mm. from the limbus. Gonin considers it most important to make these calculations accurately, even though it necessitates a delay of several days. At first he under-estimated the distance, and cauterised too close to the limbus. It is desirable to reach with the cautery, not only the anterior, but also the posterior edge of the hole. Unquestionably one reason why Gonin and his co-workers Dubois and Amsler have been so successful, is that they have with great patience and skill

accurately localised the retinal tears. Löhlein (1928) stated
that absolute localisation was rarely possible, even with a
more exact method than this. Such a determination involves
a retina in its normal position, and not one which is raised to
a varying distance from the choroid. This is a dimension that
defies absolute calculation. He therefore cauterises widely in
the affected quadrant. It is well to make sure of closing the
posterior edge of the tear as it is more efficacious to do this
than to close the anterior edge only. Gonin finds that as the
cauterisation-scar spreads during the first few weeks, a wide
choroido-retinal adhesion results. He considers recurrence
at this site impossible. It is always wise before the operation
to repeat the measurement of the distance of the tear from
the ora serrata, and the calculation of the meridian.

Now that the tear is localised, it must be projected or
orientated to its correct position on the sclera at a certain
distance behind the limbus.

PROJECTION OF A RETINAL TEAR. The finding of the point on
the sclera which corresponds with the site of the retinal tear
requires first of all the reversal of the inverted image seen by
indirect ophthalmoscopy, and then the orientation of this
erect image on to the sclera. If one draws what one sees with
indirect ophthalmoscopy, one must remember that the actual
state of the fundus is the very opposite, i.e. a feature on the
medial side is in reality on the temporal, and a tear seen at
the top of the field lies really at the bottom.

This transformation is most readily effected by rotating,
through 180 degrees, a drawing of the details in the fundus
while the paper lies flat on the table. Then one draws in the
ora serrata at the correct distance from the tear or tears. This
will represent the actual state of the details, as seen through
the pupil. To ascertain how these details will lie when we
view them from the scleral surface is the next problem. The
simplest means of solving this is by standing a plane mirror
vertically by the circular line drawn to represent the ora
serrata. The drawn details then appear on the correct side
of the ora serrata. An alternate plan is to look at the drawing
when held up to a window, and copy it on to the other side

of the paper. The final task is to estimate the distance of the tear from the limbus, as, so far, all the measurements are in disc diameters or millimetres from the ora serrata. An example of this estimation has already been given. Vogt avoids the terms "axial and peripheral" because they may be misleading. He prefers "limbusfern" and "limbusnah", for then the position of a hole is defined in terms of its distance from the limbus—the all-important landmark in ignipuncture.

If one has not been able to find the tear, one can puncture the globe at a measured distance from the limbus, and mark the scleral wound in Indian ink. This retinal puncture will be found in the fundus and if the detachment has subsided at all, it is likely that the tear will be seen. Its distance in disc diameters from the puncture can be found, and so its distance from the limbus estimated. This should be drawn and reversed to gain an erect image, and examined with a vertical mirror as described before, so that scleral projection will be accurate. Any details found at the time of operation should be entered in this drawing. The site of the operation should be marked with Indian ink. These measures may prove helpful if further operative treatment is required.

Vogt (1930) recommends the use of a special chart which can be obtained from the Ophthalmic Clinic of the University of Zurich. It consists of two triangles drawn base to base, but separated by a space 18 mm. wide. This space is divided by a central line, and where it intersects a line joining the apices of the triangles there is a peep-sight cut out of the paper. The bases of the triangles are divided into sixteen equal divisions, and lines join the apex of each triangle to the junction of these divisions. For the sake of convenience only the inner eight divisions are drawn in. The central line between the bases represents the limbus, and the sixteen divisions represent the quarters of an hour for four hours, when we are considering the limbus as the rim of a clock-face. The hours can be marked in, which correspond with the quadrant in which the tears are found. These tears can be drawn in at the correct distance from the base of the triangle, which represents the ora serrata. One holds the chart in front of the eye so that the central line, which represents the limbus, forms a tangent to the limbus at the hour which corresponds to the meridian of the tear, *i.e.* two, half-past two, or three o'clock. The line joining the apices of the triangles will then lie in this meridian. The peep-sight enables one to put the chart into the correct position. One enters the erect image of the fundus details in the triangle marked E, and copies it into the triangle marked S, by means of folding the paper and tracing the drawing through or by using a mirror and drawing in these details. The distances can be entered in ordinary figures, and Roman figures can be used for the order of the appearance of the holes or the dates of the various operations. A copy of the author's modification of Vogt's chart, and a description of the way to use it, is found in appendix (*a*) at the end of this book.

Amsler (1929) considers that the work of localisation is facilitated by using the chart of the total ophthalmoscopic field which he has used at the Lausanne University Clinic, and which he demonstrated at the 21st Annual Meeting of the Swiss Ophthalmological Society, 1928. It is a circular diagram (diameter 165 mm.; diameter of disc 5 mm.) showing the ora serrata, equator, disc and macula. On it the tear and other details of the detachment can be marked in topographically. It is divided up by concentric circles representing the ora serrata (or the most peripheral area visible ophthalmoscopically) and the equator. Six diagonals are also marked, and the twelve radii correspond to the hours of a clock. Amsler fills in on this all the essential fundus details. Next day he makes a second and independent sketch, and by comparing the two, detects any inaccuracies in the former. One must remember the possibility of several tears being present. Erggelet considers that the most exact method is to project a small beam of light through the sclera by applying the tip of an extremely narrow glass cone; Lange's lamp would serve the purpose. One then examines the fundus, and when the cone is opposite the tear, one will see a bright area. To confirm this one can switch on the lamp of the ophthalmoscope, and switch off the other lamp.

Lindner's method (1929) of projection is considerably more complicated. He seats the patient before the large

Gullstrand ophthalmoscope. The arm of a perimeter (radius 33 cm.) is attached to the ophthalmoscope, 32 cm. from the patient's cornea. On this arm a movable lamp is fixed. It enables the patient to maintain fixation of his gaze in any direction. The patient's head must remain fixed in that position which enables the observer to see the macula in the centre of the eyepiece which contains a crossed thread. The patient then follows the lamp as it is moved until the tear is in the centre of the ophthalmoscopic field. One can read off on the arm the angle between the line of central fixation and the position of the lamp when the tear is in the centre of the field. The direction of the arm is also noted. By means of a table the distance of the tear from the limbus can be ascertained. The direction of the perimetric arm gives the inclination of the tear to the horizontal line. Lindner shows that one can indicate the position of the tear in Listing's diagrammatic eye by means of a construction. He marks the horizontal meridian by a fluorescent dye applied to the edge of the cornea. He fits at the limbus a gutta-percha or metal ring of the same size as the cornea. Attached to the ring there is an adjustable indicator. Then the frame or ring is fixed in position with two conjunctival sutures. After dissecting off the conjunctiva, he places the indicator in the correct meridian, and at the corresponding distance from the limbus he marks the site for puncture. He says, "The method is only in its infancy, but it is far more exact than former methods". The main disadvantage of this method, as Lindner admits, is that the peripheral zone in which tears are so frequent is often not visible with the Gullstrand ophthalmoscope. It appears that the above contrivance is unnecessarily elaborate, and Zeiss considered that there was no need for it.[1]

CLOSING THE TEAR OR "OBLITERATING CAUTERISATION". After holocaine instillation and the injection of 2 per cent. novocaine, the conjunctiva, 3 or 4 mm. from the limbus, is divided

[1] Further information on the orientation and plotting of a fundus lesion can be obtained from papers by Tschermak (1928), Amsler and Dubois (1928), Lindner (1929), Gonin (1927), Comberg (1927), Guist (1930). Perhaps the most serviceable is that by Amsler (1929).

and a broad flap is raised. Vogt injects 1–2 c.c. of 1 per cent. cocaine and adrenalin. He prefers to operate whilst the patient is in bed, rather than on an operating table. A retrobulbar injection of at least 2 c.c. of novocaine and adrenalin will produce a proptosis and facilitate the approach to a posterior tear. The incision in the conjunctiva and the episcleral tissues should be parallel to the limbus, and the sclera should be laid bare for a distance of 1 cm. in the anteriorposterior direction, over the site of the retinal tear.

With the filled-in chart before one, one marks the limbus, with methylene blue, at the two points where the meridian of the tear crosses it. At the point remote from the tear, one inserts a fine silk suture knotted at its end, so that it will not pull through. One draws the thread across the other point, and over the bare sclera. This demonstrates the line of the meridian and it is marked in in Indian ink or methylene blue. Then using a sterilised steel tape, or calipers, one measures the distance along this line that corresponds with the distance of the tear from the limbus. One marks this point with methylene blue or gentian violet. Vogt advises the marking of the meridian prior to the incision of the conjunctiva. He uses a fine needle and silk for the sutures.

Rubbrecht (1929) temporarily divides the horizontal rectus muscle that is closest to the site of the tear. A thread is put through the two ends of the muscle and tied at the end of the operation. The insertion of the muscle enables an assistant to fix the globe firmly with forceps. This tenotomy appears unnecessary.[1]

All bleeding must be arrested as this may obscure one's landmarks. The thread can be removed when the sclera is marked, for the operator is accurately orientated. The sclera is opened in this line, layer by layer, with a Graefe knife. Vogt inserts the knife with its back towards the posterior pole of the eye, and cutting away from the sclera makes an incision from 1 to 3 mm. in length. Others make an incision twice as long

---

[1] Schoenberg (1930) has pointed out that there is considerable danger of injuring important structures during the ignipuncture. A summary of the chief landmarks in the Topographical Anatomy of the Eyeball is given in Appendix b.

(Rubbrecht). They hold that a long incision is indicated because of the possibility of error in calculating the distance, and because of the need of including both edges of the rent in the cauterisation. One must remember that the edges may be 1·5 mm. or more apart. In a triangular tear, the base may be 3 or 4 mm. from the summit. With a larger incision there is a greater danger of losing the more solid vitreous, and this should be avoided. Amsler makes an incision only $1\frac{1}{2}$ mm. in length, and the anterior extremity of it corresponds with the scleral landmark which shows the site of the tear. The centre of the incision must be from $\frac{1}{2}$ to 1 mm. posterior to the tear. "Une cautérisation trop postérieure est encore utile; elle fait barrage; trop antérieure, elle ne sert à rien" (Coppez). The limit that one can reach on the nasal side appears to be 22 mm. from the limbus. In the inferior temporal quadrant one can go a little further. If one loses sight of the incision, it is wiser to find it with a small strabismus hook than by probing with the cautery. A Desmarres retractor is of value for the protection of the conjunctiva and the lid. The Graefe knife need not be inserted further than is necessary to perforate the choroid. A slight rotation of the knife will enable some of the subretinal fluid to escape. The knife is then withdrawn and when the fluid ceases to flow a Paquelin or a galvano-cautery with a hook-shaped end at red heat is used without delay. Gonin uses a Paquelin with a specially small tip ($\frac{1}{2}$ mm. at the point) at white heat. He inserts it into the wound to a depth of 2 or 3 mm. and cauterises for two or three seconds. This burns the neighbouring sclera and choroid, and the retina, if it comes in contact with the tip of the cautery, adheres to it. The cauterisation produces a burn, which as it heals unites firmly the three coats of the eye and probably the vitreous in a cicatrix. Vogt also prefers a cautery at white heat (about 1000° C. while red heat is about 500° C.). If there is an abundant flow of vitreous, only a white hot cautery will prove effective. Von Hippel (1929) considered that his failure to close the tears in four detachments was due to the fact that he used a cautery just glowing instead of red or white hot. Vogt inserts only 1–2 mm. of the tip of the cautery through the scleral wound. He has at times cauterised under the guidance of the ophthalmoscope—a procedure which must be most difficult. He has found that too prolonged a cauterisation, or the insertion of the cautery too far into the eye, may produce a white opacity in the affected area of vitreous. If the cautery cannot be drawn away because it has become adherent to the coagulated tissues, one must cauterise further, until, with slight traction, it comes away.

The conjunctival wound must be closed with sutures. Both eyes are tied up and dressed on the fifth day. From then on, atropine is inserted daily. The patient is allowed up on the ninth or tenth day. Vogt, however, allows his patients to get out of bed and have a short walk on the day after the operation. From then on, he allows them to be up daily for from two to four hours. It is wise to adjust the position of the head in bed so that, if possible, the vitreous will press down on the cauterised area.

One should rarely attempt to cauterise two tears at one operation. If one fails to close a tear, it is wise to cauterise it again before attempting to close a second tear. "Il faut corriger son tir" (Gonin). Gonin stated (1928): "If it is evident that a mistake has been made in calculating, and that the tear is still visible in the vicinity of the operation scar, then, as in artillery firing, the first wrong shot can be corrected by altering elevation and side as required for the second shot. This is practically a mathematical process, and I have never required to make a correction more than once for one and the same tear, excepting in cases where the rupture was so great that it was obvious from the beginning that it would not be closed with a single scar". If the tear is opposite a muscle, it is usually sufficient to draw it aside, but it may be necessary to make a buttonhole in it by means of a longitudinal incision and cauterise through this. Gonin says: "In spite of every care and precision, it is still uncertain of course, whether the desired spot in the retina has been touched, and whether the opening will be completely closed by the scar. One can only be certain after six or seven days". Both Gonin and Vogt cauterise through the sclera itself at times. Vogt finds this of value, especially if the tear is situated at a great distance from the limbus. He then uses the galvano-cautery. Sometimes, if there is a series of holes or several large holes in one area, he cauterises superficially a considerable area of the sclera surrounding the site of the hole. He makes multiple punctures of the scleral surface over an area 3–4 mm. square. Then he perforates the sclera, and makes the ignipuncture. This superficial cauterisation may enable one to close a series of holes at one operation. The essential difference between this operation and the older operation of cautery-puncture, is that now the operation is done in the actual neighbourhood of the tear.

Vogt considers that one is justified in attempting to close large rents or two adjacent holes by ignipunctures at two sites at one sitting, if the patient can rotate the eye unaided into a convenient position. If one has to force the eye by traction with forceps, the risk of vitreous loss is too great. It can be taken as a general rule that the less the movement of the eye, especially if forced, the less will be the risk of vitreous loss, the degree of heat required, and the duration of the operation. The rotation of the eye by an assistant is, however, at times unavoidable, especially if the tear is in the upper and nasal areas. For a temporal tear, situated at a considerable distance from the limbus, Krönlein's operation may be a useful preliminary. Vogt's protective spoon may be of advantage in an operation if the tear is posterior to the equator. For varying circumstances, a varied series of such spoons is necessary for keeping an unimpeded view of the sclera, by pressing away the orbital contents. They are from 1 to 1½ cm. in breadth and can be bent as required. Pressure on the globe must be avoided. For such conditions the loop of the cautery must be so bent that the sclera is touched only at the desired point. With such instruments one can open the sclera even at the posterior pole.

Vogt considers that it is wise to cauterise all perforating wounds of the sclera which involve the vitreous. By so doing we lessen the risk of detachment and even if a detachment does occur in such a case Vogt considers that the cauterisation may lead to its re-attachment. He considers that the tear is the essential lesion in the majority of such cases.

Gonin considers that success will follow an operation only

if the tear is included in the scar. Vogt and Wessely each report a cure where a tear had not been found. This, however, is not to be anticipated, and all means to find a tear or tears should be taken. After cauterisation the punctured area in the fundus will appear white with a certain degree of surrounding or overlying pigmentation. In this area the retina and the vitreous are adherent to the choroid and the sclera.

RESULTS OF TREATMENT. In this brief résumé of Gonin's work, it is well to keep in mind the conclusion arrived at six years ago by one of the leading oculists of the English-speaking world: "Personally I have seen no case in which there was a hole, improved either spontaneously or after treatment, and it is my opinion that, with our present available methods, such cases of detachment are practically hopeless" (Sir William Lister, 1924). This attitude and the apparent grossness of the method advocated for the closure of a minute hole in a delicate nervous tissue make one incredulous when one first hears of Gonin's operation. As Vogt wrote: "Every opthalmologist will shake his head when he hears of such an operation. 'How', he will ask, 'can such a drastic method as cauterisation cause the closing up of a tear in such a fragile and delicate membrane as the retina, when it might even be the cause of detachment of the retina in a healthy eye? Is it not as bad as shooting sparrows with a cannon?'"

In 1928, when publishing eight fresh cures, Gonin stated that to the five cures amongst ten detachments reported in his previous communication, one more might be added. The vision of a sixth patient had in the interval improved from 1/150 to 1/10. In this instance he had operated five months after the lesion had developed. The tear was a large rent at the ora serrata. The five other re-attachments were unchanged. The eight detachments being reported for the first time were, with one exception, in myopic patients. Two of these patients had had cataract extractions prior to the development of the detachment. One of these showed an almost complete detachment of three months' duration. It became re-attached, and eight months after operation it was still classed as a cure. Another patient had a detachment with a large tear and another one showed two tears. He reported partial cures in two patients with numerous retinal tears.

Gonin wrote (1928 a): "In my more recent attempts at operative closing of retinal tears, I succeeded twenty-six times in definitely and completely closing up a small tear (1–2 P.D.) with a single cauterisation, and on three occasions the same scar also closed up a second tear in its immediate vicinity. Only five times had a fault in localising to be corrected subsequently. Of the large ruptures (3–5 P.D. or more), four closed up after a second hot-needle puncture; in two of them three punctures were needed, and in two others four punctures were required to make the adhesion-scar complete".

Vogt (1928–9), though he at first looked with scepticism at this operation, is now an ardent supporter of it. He was surprised at the splendid results that he obtained in three extensive long-standing retinal detachments. His first and experimental case was as follows: A boy, aged seventeen years, who two years before, as a result of an injury with a stone, developed a complete detachment of the retina. After five months' treatment in hospital along conservative lines, his vision was barely 0·1. Two years after the onset, Vogt was able to cauterise the retinal hole, and within fourteen days it was closed. Eighteen months later, his vision was = 1. The time which elapsed before operation enabled the retina and the hole, which had been at a considerable distance from the choroid, to settle down and come more within range.

His second patient was a female patient with 5 D. of myopia. A spontaneous detachment had developed in February 1927. After three months of conservative measures, including saline injections by other oculists, Vogt cauterised in July 1927. Vision increased from 0·1 to 0·7. Here again the retinal tear had come closer to the choroid during the interval before operation. In December 1928, this patient was re-examined when a smooth white scar was found in the fundus, and vision was still 0·7.

The third patient was a woman, aged thirty, with 4 D. of myopia. After six months of treatment by conservative measures, a cauterisation of the hole was done. The hole was closed, and vision improved from 0·1 to 0·7. Sixteen months later it was unchanged. This brief survey of these patients shows that this method of treatment can succeed in very difficult cases and in those that hitherto have been inoperable.

Vogt describes various types of distorted vision as a result of the reapplication of the macula. There may be a "restlessness" of the central area of the visual field. Not only has the applied layer of cones to make new relationships with the retinal epithelium, but it has also to recover from the interference with nutrition due to its detachment. It is astonishing that this recovery can occur after detachment of many months' duration. Vogt describes the return of full visual acuity when a detachment had been present for more than eight months. Such observations certainly disprove the idea that specific relationships exist for any individual cone and the corresponding epithelial cells. In re-attachment, it is impossible that each cone returns to its original position. Visual acuity may steadily improve during the first few months after reapplication. The retinal reflexes seen so clearly with red-free light may take several months to disappear. The development of a mild oedema of the disc after re-attachment due to ignipuncture has been observed (Vogt, 1930).

Vogt states that it is not necessary to touch the hole directly. If one cauterises within one or two D.D. it is sufficient. If the cauterisation is still farther from the hole, the cure may not ensue for several months. Certain pictures which he has published of fundi after cauterisation certainly show holes that have been closed merely by a cauterisation in the vicinity. In some, the scar appeared to be from one to two disc diameters away. If the cauterisation were further away, there is a possibility that the hole may close during the subsequent few months. Vogt reports a male, aged forty-five, with a large semi-lunar hole 1½ P.D. in width, and situated temporally 8 P.D. from the disc. He had had other treatment for six months. The cautery was applied 2 P.D. too high, and only the upper lip of the hole became re-attached at the time. However, six months later he reported that his vision was almost normal. In four other patients he cauterised without finding a hole, and little benefit resulted. Later he stated that it was useless to make an ignipuncture unless a tear had been found (1929a).

Vogt reports three patients treated by him, in whom the tear in the retina was at a considerable distance from the choroid. In none of these did complete closure follow even repeated cauterisation. He considers that it may be advisable to wait, and by conservative measures attempt to lessen the subretinal fluid, and so bring the retina closer to the choroid.

One detachment reported by Vogt shows that occasionally a retina may be so degenerate that further tears continue to appear. This lowered resistance accounts for a proportion of the failures in series reported even by Vogt and Gonin. One patient who was treated successfully by Vogt introduced an interesting point. The left eye was emmetropic and the retina and vitreous normal. The other eye was myopic and the retina had become detached during gymnastics. As this eye had been divergent it had therefore not been subjected to any of the excessive near work which is often stressed as a cause of the presenile degeneration so characteristic of myopia. However, the customary lesions were present. Vogt claimed that myopia *per se* and not excessive near work explained such degeneration.

Vogt considers that the following points are still undecided: the most suitable duration of time for cauterisation, the best temperature, the most suitable depth to insert the cautery and whether a hot needle is preferable to a cautery. He concludes that "these and other unanswered questions are intended merely to guard us from exaggerated optimism which is a danger of every new method. For the present we can be satisfied with the surprising results in cases which, without Gonin's idea, would have been as good as lost".

To show the determination necessary on the part of the operator and patient alike, one can refer to Vogt's patient (1930) (No. 7) who had had conservative treatment for retinal detachment for seven months. She was aged forty-six, and a myope of 4 D. At first no tear could be found, but after repeated examinations three suspicious areas were seen. By the end of a year's treatment, during which time four ignipunctures had been carried out, the condition of the detachment was definitely worse. Hand movements could just be detected, and the retina was grey-green and completely detached. At last, however, a tear could be seen. This was cauterised, and the retina re-attached completely. This was twenty-one months after the onset of the detachment. Six weeks after this operation the vision was 5/15.

An apparent success which, if permanent, is a triumph, was made in treating an almost complete detachment showing eleven tears in a myopic eye (− 16 D.) (No. 11). The other eye was quite blind from a detachment which had developed fourteen years before. Eight days after vision failed, seven retinal rents were found. These were mainly in an area between 12 and 3 o'clock and from 3–5 D.D. from the ora serrata. After two operations when the patient had had a fifteen minutes' walk, a partial recurrence was found. Four more tears were found, but after four more operations at intervals of one, three, and five weeks, the retina was completely re-attached, and the visual field full. Ten weeks after discharge the vision was as sharp as it had been before the detachment developed.

Another patient who had an unfavourable prognosis, and was treated successfully, was a forty-six-year-old myopic albino (No. 14). She had a detachment with a very large hole (3 D.D. in diameter) and situated 5–6 D.D. from the disc in the superior temporal quadrant. This hole had a small lid which moved as the eye was rotated. The two unfavourable points were the size of the hole and its great distance from the limbus. The first ignipuncture was made at a distance of 15 mm. from the limbus, but only the upper edge of the hole re-attached. In order to cauterise further back, a special protective retractor was made to press away the orbital contents from the site of operation. A platinum cautery with a bent end, and longer than usual, was pressed on the sclera many times. The hole closed after this, but a second hole would require closing by a second operation before this detachment could be classed as a cure.

Vogt reports the appearance of small grey areas which he considered to be the lids of holes. They can completely or only partially hide the holes from view. Two were found in a patient (No. 15) who had had a detachment for three months. They were 1/4–1/5 D.D. in diameter, and one showed a definite parallax with the hole which it only partially hid. These holes were closed. Afterwards for a period of some weeks a greyish veil was noticed in front of one of the scarred holes.

A woman, aged thirty-one, with 5½ D. of myopia is reported, who, having lost the vision in one eye from detachment, eight years before, developed a similar condition in her other eye. Eight months after the onset, and after an ignipuncture had been performed without permanent benefit by another surgeon, Vogt found an extensive detachment showing a series of nine holes in a small area, 3½ D.D. from the ora serrata. They faded into an area showing cystoid degeneration. After a single ignipuncture the retina reattached completely, and after four and a half months the vision was = 1.

Arruga (1929) confirms Gonin's findings. He considers that the finding and the localising of the tears constitute the greatest difficulties. He states that 50 per cent. of detachments can be healed if they are recent, and have not previously been treated in any other way, and if the tears are small and near the equator. This percentage is reduced to ten, if one or two months have elapsed since the onset, if the tears are large, multiple or post-equatorial, or if extensive retino-choroidal changes are present. Practically no case is cured if the tears are inaccessible because they cannot be found, or because they are situated in the region of the macula. Tears with ragged edges appeared to be the most difficult to close. Lindner (1929 b–30) described eleven patients whom he had treated by this method. He burns through the sclera layer by layer, and then punctures the choroid with the cold galvano-cautery. Then the current is turned on, and the point is left in the wound for from ten to twenty seconds. The eye is not examined for from eight to fourteen days. He had found tears in fourteen of the last twenty-one patients he had seen. In two, the holes were macular. One tear he had considered too large to justify interference, but because of his success with Gonin's method, he would now operate. One of his patients with a detachment of six weeks' duration showed a long tear. He cauterised first one side of the tear, then the other, and then the centre, applying the cautery for fifteen seconds each time. Vision was improved to 6/9. Of the eight detachments that he has treated by ignipuncture, seven appeared to be permanent cures. Three had vision of 6/9, and two of 6/18. That the technique had not been perfected is shown in one case in which five attempts were made before the tear was successfully cured. The final vision was 6/36. Siegrist (1928) considers that ignipuncture is the best and most successful operation. He first sent his patients to Gonin for treatment. However, when he saw how good the results were, he acquired the technique, and has met with considerable success. A few weeks after operating on his first case the hole was completely healed. Seefelder (1929) had success in treating detachments in which no tear could be found. In all his patients, repeated punctures had been necessary. Of five patients, one was completely cured, another almost so, and two showed improved vision and arrest of the detachment. Stock (1929) reports thirteen detachments operated on by this method. Two were hopeless from the start, and two others were considered unsuitable for operation. Of the remaining nine, six showed no improvement. The three remaining detachments were successfully treated, and Stock is of the opinion that more success can be attained by this method than by any other. Pincus (1929) reported a test case which he sent to Gonin for treatment. An engineer, aged forty, whose right eye had been blind for twenty years from detachment of the retina, noticed disquieting symptoms in the lower part of his left visual field. A very flat detachment was found, but neither Pincus nor his colleague found a tear. However, even though his vision was 6/6, when 10 D. of myopia and 2 D. of astigmatism were corrected, Gonin, on finding a small tear, cauterised it. It was healed, and a full field was restored. This is a demonstration of Gonin's ability. It was an only eye, with 6/6 vision, and a tear in an unfavourable position, and yet he did not hesitate to carry out his usual treatment.

Igersheimer (1929) reports an only eye with a total

detachment showing a large tear. He considered it hopeless. However, at the first attempt he completely closed the tear even though it was considerably larger than the cauterised area. After reporting seven cases treated in this way, he concludes that Gonin's operation is a great forward step, but that "ablatio retinae" still remains a serious malady. Weill (1929) refers to twelve patients with detachment, five of whom were treated according to Gonin's method. He was unable to reach the tear at the first attempt, as a rule. Wessely (1929) was inclined to consider that many of the cures were only temporary. Gradle reported (1930) his early experiences with this method, and they were certainly not encouraging. He, however, is satisfied that "within the space of one year there have been more reliable reports of cures of retinal detachments than all other methods have accomplished in more than ten years". Brückner (1929) reported five complete cures amongst twelve patients treated by Gonin's method. The cures had been watched for from three to six months only after operation.

These reports emphasise the difficulty of finding and localising the tear in the majority of cases. To obtain success, strict adherence to Gonin's technique is essential. If one fails it must be one's technique rather than Gonin's operation that receives the blame until one's method is above suspicion. Careful consideration of each case on its own merits must always be made. Not all detachments are due to retinal tears. As Pascheff (1929) has already reminded us "there are cases of detachment without a tear, and cases of spontaneous healing, and in the latter a choroidal lesion is usually to blame". It appears that ignipuncture acts not only by sealing the hole, and so restoring the conditions which make for a preretinal pressure in excess of that in the inter-retinal space, but also by reproducing the inflammatory lesion, which probably explains the tendency for fluid to absorb, and thus the better prognosis in those detachments which are due to exudation.

REFERENCES

PROPHYLACTIC TREATMENT

1922. STARGARDT, K. *Klin. Monatsbl. f. Augenheilk.* **68**, 826.
1924. GUIBERT. *Clin. Ophtal.* **28**, 438.
1928. GRUNERT, K. *Klin. Monatsbl. f. Augenheilk.* **80**, 522.
1928. VOGT, A. *Ibid.* **80**, 709.
1929. BIRCH-HIRSCHFELD. *Zeitschr. f. Augenheilk.* **68**, 127.
1929. MELLER, J. *Klin. Monatsbl. f. Augenheilk.* **83**, 821.
1929. ANKLESARIA, M. D. *Indian Med. Gaz.* April, **64**, 186.

DRUGS

1921. LAMB, R. S. and ZIEGLER. *Amer. Jl. of Ophthal.* **4**, 668.
1921. VIGANO, E. V. *Jl. Amer. Med. Assoc.* (abstract), **77**, 110.
1928. KERRY, R. *Canad. M.A.J.* **18**, 62.
1928. HAMBURGER, C. *Münch. med. Wochenschr.* **75**, 52, 2208.
1929. ASCHNER, B. *Ibid.* Dec. 2135.
1929. JABLONSKI, W. *Ibid.* **76**, 42, 1762.
1929. KERRY, R. *Brit. Jl. of Ophthal.* **13**, 447.

COMPRESSION BANDAGE

1875. SAMELSOHN. *Zentralbl. f. d. med. Wiss.* **49**, 833.
1887. —— *Zentralbl. f. p. Augenheilk.* **11**, 351.
1905. WESSELY, K. *Klin. Monatsbl. f. Augenheilk.* **43**, Part 1, 654.
1920. MENDOZA. *Clin. Ophtal.* **24**, 545.
1921. GONIN, J. *Ann. d'Ocul.* **158**, 175.
1922. MAGITOT, A. P. and BAILLIART, P. *Amer. Jl. of Ophthal.* **5**, 824.
1922. WESSELY, K. *Klin. Monatsbl. f. Augenheilk.* **68**, 275.
1929. SCHMELZER, R. *Arch. of Ophthal.* **1**, 113.

DIET

1922. MARX, E. *Arch. f. Ophthal.* **108**, 237.
1922. STARGARDT, K. *Zeitschr. f. Augenheilk.* **48**, 161.
1922. TRISTAINO, B. *Gior. di Ocul. Naples*, **3**, 109.
1923. NOISZEWSKI. *Klin. Monatsbl. f. Augenheilk.* **71**, 271.
1924. ROCHAT and STEIJN. *Brit. Jl. of Ophthal.* **8**, 257.

OPERATIVE TREATMENT

THE FORMATION OF ADHESIONS

1805. WARE, JAMES. *Chirurg. Observ. relat. to the Eye*, **2**, 238.
1860. HANCOCK, H. *Ophthal. Hosp. Rep. London*, **3**, 13.
1863. V. GRAEFE, A. *Arch. f. Ophthal.* **9**, 85.
1881. DE WECKER. *Ann. d'Ocul.* **87**, 39.

1882. ABADIE, C. *Gaz. hedb.* 49.
1890. GALEZOWSKI. *Recueil d'ophtal.* 1.
1894. SCHEFFELS. *Michel's Jahresber.* 415.
1895. DOR, H. *Bull. et Mém. Soc. franç. d'Ophtal.* **13**, 181.
1906. WERNICKE, G. *Klin. Monatsbl. f. Augenheilk.* **44**, 1, 134.
1907. DOR, H. *Bull. et Mém. Soc. franç. d'Ophtal.* **24**, 342.
1907. DOR, L. *Ann. d'Ocul.* **137**, 440.
1923. HANDMANN. *Klin. Monatsbl. f. Augenheilk.* **71**, 222.
1923. SOURDILLE, G. *Arch. d'Ophtal.* **40**, 419.
1924. WIENER, MEYER. *Arch. of Ophthal.* **53**, 368.
1925. WALKER. *Ibid.* **54**, 562.
1926. GALLOIS, J. *Bull. Soc. d'Ophtal. de Paris*, April, 158.
1928. THIEL. *Ber. über der deutsch. ophth. Gesell.* Heidelberg, 50.
1929. SOURDILLE, G. *Prat. Med. franç.*
1929. MARTIN. *Elschnig. Augenaertz. Operat.* **2**, 701.

ELECTROLYSIS

1895. CLAVELIER and MARAVEL. *Ann. d'Ocul.* **115**, 37.
1895. TERSON. *Ibid.* **114**, 22.
1896. SNELL, S. *Trans. Ophthal. Soc. U.K.* **16**, 72.
1896. MONTGOMERY. *Jl. Amer. Med. Assoc.* **27**, 702.
1897. LAGRANGE. *Ann. d'Ocul.* **118**, 47.
1897. CLAVELIER. *Michel's Jahresber.* 512.
1901. MARAVEL. *Clin. Ophtal.* 260.
1930. STALLARD. *Brit Jl. of Ophthal.* **14**, 1.

SUBCONJUNCTIVAL INJECTIONS

1896. MELLINGER. *Jahresber. der Augenheilk. in Basel*, **32**, 82.
1896. DOR, H. *Bull. et Mém. Soc. franç. d'Ophtal.* **14**, 396.
1906. RAMSAY, A. MAITLAND. *Trans. Ophthal. Soc. U.K.* **26**, 79.
1915. MARQUEZ. *Arch. de Oftal. Hisp. Amer.* 478.
1920. DARIER, A. *Clin. Ophtal.* **9**, 10.
1921. MOORE, R. FOSTER. *Lancet*, July, 174.
1922. TERRIEN, F. *Jl. Amer. Med. Assoc.* **78**, 848.
1922. HERKEL, E. B. *Amer. Jl. of Ophthal.* **5**, 563.
1922. TRISTAINO, B. *Gior. di Ocul. Naples*, **3**, 109.
1930. STALLARD, H. B. *Brit. Jl. of Ophthal.* **14**, 11.

THE DIVISION OF VITREOUS STRANDS

1895. DEUTSCHMANN, R. *Klin. Monatsbl. f. Augenheilk.* **51**, 762.
1930.   —— *Münch. med. Wochenschr.* **77**, 102.

THE REDUCTION OF OCULAR CAPACITY

1920. TÖRÖKE. *Arch. of Ophthal.* **49**, 506.
1927. KOCH, C. *Klin. Monatsbl. f. Augenheilk.* **79**, 138.

THE PROVISION OF PERMANENT DRAINAGE

1872. DE WECKER. *Ann. d'Ocul.* Sept. 137.
1873. ROBERTSON, ARGYLL. *Ophthal. Hosp. Rep. London*, **8**, 3, 404.
1890. GALEZOWSKI, X. *Recueil d'Ophtal.* **3**, 1.
1915. PARKER. *Sect. Ophthal. Amer. Med. Assoc.* 106.
1916. THOMSON, E. S. and CURTIN. *Jl. Amer. Med. Assoc.* April, 330.
1919. OHM. *Deut. med. Wochenschr.* **43**, 748.
1920. THOMSON, E. S. and CURTIN. *Arch. of Ophthal.* **49**, 563.
1921. CHIPMAN, L. *Canad. M.A.J.* **10**, 1007.
1921. DAMEL, C. S. *Semana Med.* April, 478.
1921. GROENHOLM, V. *Arch. f. Ophthal.* **105**, 899.
1923. MELLER, J. *Ophthal. Surgery*, 3rd edn., trans. by Sweet, 311.
1923. LAMBERT. *Arch. of Ophthal.* **52**, 267.
1924. HESSBERG. *Zeitschr. f. Augenheilk.* **53**, 118.
1924. WIENER, MEYER. *Arch. of Ophthal.* **53**, 368.
1926. MACCALLAN. *Amer. Jl. of Ophthal.* Ser. 3, **9**, 455.
1926. SLOAN. *Southern med. Jl.* 228.
1928. LA FERLA, O. A. *Boll. d'Ocul.* **7**, 142.

THE RAISING OF THE INTRA-OCULAR TENSION

1912. LAGRANGE, R. *Rev. gén. d'Ophtal.* **31**, 379.
1912. ROHMER. *Arch. d'Ophtal.* **32**, May, 257.
1920. WOOD, D. J. *Brit. Jl. of Ophthal.* **4**, 413.
1921. PESME. *Arch. d'Ophtal.* **38**, Oct.
1921. WIEDEN, E. *Rev. Cubana de Oft.* **3**, 680.
1922. STARGARDT, K. *Klin. Monatsbl. f. Augenheilk.* **68**, 826.
1923. DELORME. *Arch. d'Ophtal.* **40**, 166.
1923. LÖWENSTEIN, A. *Klin. Monatsbl. f. Augenheilk.* **71**, 769.
1923. DEL CASTILLO. *Arch. de Oftal. Hisp. Amer.* **23**, 521.
1924. CARBONE. *Soc. Ital. di Oftal.* 301.
1925. VITOU. *Clin. Ophtal.* 2nd. ser. **14**, 54.
1926. VAN HEUVEN. *Klin. Monatsbl. f. Augenheilk.* **76**, 136, 340.
1926. PROKSCH, M. *Ibid.* **76**, 133.
1926. NAKASHIMA, M. *Arch. f. Ophthal.* **117**, 403.
1926. JEANDELIZE, P. and BAUDOT, R. *Arch. d'Ophtal.* **43**, 413.
1928. CSAPODY, J. *Klin. Monatsbl. f. Augenheilk.* **80**, 641.
1928. BIRCH-HIRSCHFELD. *Ibid.* **80**, 531.
1928. BETTREMIEUX. *Ann. d'Ocul.* **165**, 914.
1929. —— *Arch. d'Ophtal.* **46**, 285.
1929. V. RÖTTH. *Klin. Monatsbl. f. Augenheilk.* **83**, 359.
1929. FODER, G. *Ibid.* **83**, 360.

IGNIPUNCTURE, OR GONIN'S METHOD OF TREATMENT

1920. JOCQS, R. *Clin. Ophtal.* **9**, 357.
1921. GONIN, J. *Ann. d'Ocul.* **158**, 175.
1924. LISTER, Sir WM. *Brit. Jl. of Ophthal.* **8**, 19.

1927. COMBERG, W. *Arch. f. Ophthal.* **118,** 175.
1927. GONIN, J. *Arch. d'Ophtal.* Sept. **44,** 560.
1927. —— *Ann. d'Ocul.* **163,** 817.
1927. —— *Arch. f. Ophthal.*
1928. —— *Ber. ü. d. Versamml. d. deutsch. ophthal. Gesellsch.* **74,** 46, 445.
1928. VOGT, A. *Klin. Monatsbl. f. Augenheilk.* **81,** 708.
1928 a. GONIN, J. *Ber. ü. d. Versamml. d. deutsch. ophthal. Gesellsch.* **74,** 46.
1928 b. —— *Arch. d'Ophtal.* **45,** 554.
1928. AMSLER, M. *Ber. ü. d. Versamml. d. deutsch. ophthal. Gesellsch.* **74,** 50.
1928. TSCHERMAK, A. *Ibid.* **74,** 33.
1928. AMSLER, M. and DUBOIS, H. *Klin. Monatsbl. f. Augenheilk.* **80,** 710.
1928. SIEGRIST, A. *Ibid.* **81,** 708.
1928. LÖHLEIN. *Ber. ü. d. Versamml. d. deutsch. ophthal. Gesellsch.* **74,** 51.
1929 a. VOGT, A. *Klin. Monatsbl. f. Augenheilk.* (5th patient), **82,** 626.
1929 b. —— *Schweiz med. Wochenschr.* March, 331.
1929. RUBBRECHT, R. *Bull. de Soc. belge d'Ophtal.* **59,** 15.
1929. AMSLER, M. *Bull. de Soc. d'Ophtal. de Paris,* **9,** 17.
1929. IGERSHEIMER; WEILL; BRUCKNER, Z.; PASCHEFF, C.; PINCUS. *Klin. Monatsbl. f. Augenheilk.* **83,** 668.
1929. WESSELY, C.; SEEFELDER, R.; VON HIPPEL, E. *Ibid.* **83,** 331.
1929 a. LINDNER, K. *Ibid.* **82,** 119; *Arch. f. Ophthal.* **123,** 234.
1929 b. —— *Klin. Monatsbl. f. Augenheilk.* **83,** 679.
1929. ARRUGA. *Arch. de Oftal. Hisp. Amer.* **29,** 346; abstract in *Klin. Monatsbl. f. Augenheilk.* **83,** 852.
1929. STOCK. *Klin. Monatsbl. f. Augenheilk.* **83,** 353.
1929. SALZMANN, M. *Arch. f. Ophthal.* **123,** 252.
1930. VOGT, A. *Klin. Monatsbl. f. Augenheilk.* **84,** 305.
1930. GRADLE, H. S. *Amer. Jl. of Ophthal.* **13,** 304.
1930. GUIST, G.; LINDNER, K. "Zeiss, Carl", *Klin. Monatsbl. f. Augenheilk.* **84,** 120.
1930. SCHOENBERG, M. J. *Arch. of Ophthal.* **3,** June 1930, 684.

CHAPTER VI

PROGNOSIS

SPONTANEOUS RE-ATTACHMENT. The first question that we must consider is that of spontaneous re-attachment. Leber describes the various manners in which this may occur, sometimes rapidly, and at other times very gradually; sometimes during rest and conservative treatment, and at times when no treatment was being carried out. Rarely is the cure as dramatic as one described by de Schweinitz (1899). In his patient the detachment was complete and of almost three months' duration. After forty-eight hours of absolute rest, the retina became completely re-attached. Vision was 20/70, and the field was full, but the duration of this recovery was not stated. Several strange instances have been described of re-attachment occurring during or after falls or violent movements, such as during vomiting (Remak, 1907; Mooren, 1882). Others have described detachments which have alternately attached and detached as many as five times (Stilling, 1883; Hirschberg, 1874). Leber considered that this could occur only if a tear were present. Horstmann (1898), Schweigger (1883), Hirschberg (1891), Leber and Frankel (1895) described thirteen detachments which behaved in this manner. These were mainly in middle-aged myopes, and appeared to be permanent. Leber observed one of his patients, a myope of 14·0 D., aged fifty-four, for twenty-five years. A detachment reported by Highett (1924) cleared up seven days after a sudden onset, only to recur five weeks later. After a month it disappeared, and two months later reappeared; five weeks later it had completely vanished. Three and a half months later the fundi was still normal. The only treatment was rest in bed, a lightly applied bandage, and the instillation of 5 per cent. dionine. No tear was found.

More recently Birch-Hirschfeld stated that 1 per cent. of detachments cleared up spontaneously. Ernest Thomson, however, stated that it was as high as 7·2 per cent. and that after all forms of treatment it was only 10 per cent. Souter refers to six spontaneous cures (1927). Two were traumatic in origin, one myopic, and one associated with pregnancy, whilst no cause was found in two others. In three, atrophic changes were left behind, in two retinal striae, and in one the fundus appeared normal. Fisher (1916) reported four detachments which recovered spontaneously. He considered choroidal exudate to be the cause, and its absorption the means of cure. In a highly myopic child, aged twelve, he had found a detachment which produced a scotoma. This scotoma gradually grew smaller and ascended in the visual field as the exudate descended. It disappeared after several months. Six years later a transparent localised detachment appeared in the other eye. After two months this could not be seen. No relapse took place during the following nine years. Killen (1916) reported an example of spontaneous recovery which was similar in some ways to this. A myope, aged thirty-five, developed a detachment, which disappeared after a fortnight's conservative treatment. It returned a few days later, and after a journey by rail and sea it again disappeared. It, however, soon returned, but after some weeks of rest and treatment with pilocarpine and subconjunctival saline it subsided. When a detachment developed some years later, in the other eye, it disappeared during a course of similar treatment. Fisher reported another patient who, when making an unexpected recovery from an illness of pyaemic character, developed a detachment which gradually subsided. Two years later the visual field was still full. That spontaneous recovery is a possibility if exudate has caused the detachment is shown by a second patient described by Killen. A myopic male, aged fifty-three, developed a detachment in an eye in which six months before areas regarded as choroiditis were found.

If one included puerperal cases, a much larger percentage would be described (Kraus (1924), Benedict and Mussey (1923), Fry (1929), Gardner (1923), Schiötz (1921), Clapp (1919), Hill (1924) and many others). In some of the eyes, the detachments recurred at the following pregnancy. In a patient reported by Schiötz, the recurrence was after an interval of five years. However, after abortion, the retina became re-attached. From a study of this form of detachment, one must admit that the longer the interval between the onset of the detachment and the termination of pregnancy, the smaller the chances of re-attachment. In another patient reported by Schiötz no retinitis was present, and the detachment appeared to be permanent. This is a rare finding. It must not be forgotten that the association of the two conditions, pregnancy and detachment of the retina, may only be accidental. Schiötz refers to the description of five such detachments in the literature. Of these, three of the patients were highly myopic. If, in the absence of nephritis, a detachment appears, it must be considered "idiopathic" in type, requiring the usual treatment and with the same bad prognosis. Heine (1929) considers that the presence of a detachment suggests a chronic nephritis, and so makes the outlook more serious than a mild retinitis. It is therefore a more definite indication for interrupting pregnancy.

Some detachments seem to reach a certain stage and become stationary. A patient described by Neame (1928) showed a detachment which was unchanged for seventeen years, and the vision remained at 6/18. This, however, is very exceptional. The undoubted tendency is to complete separation and then the retina assumes the form of a convolvulus flower (Arlt). It loses its grey appearance, and becomes transparent again. At one stage, the beam of the slit-lamp will become apparent at the detached retina and again on the choroid, but when the retina is atrophic and transparent, the former area of light tends to fade.

Complete recovery of vision is probably aided by the ability of the retinal epithelium to proliferate and spread. In addition these cells may have the amoeboid tendencies exhibited by them in the lower animals. There is also a tendency for the lamina vitrea to form a hyaline substance which too may aid in re-attachment. Disintegration of the rods and cones and the external limiting membrane and probably other changes excite proliferation of this tissue in man.

THE EFFECT OF A RETINAL TEAR. It is probable that the majority of spontaneous re-attachments occur when choroidal effusion has been the primary lesion. It is difficult to understand a cure following the dragging due to vitreous strands. The part played by retinal tears in such eyes is difficult to decide. Leber considered that a hole was essential, if one was to get re-attachment. He hoped that the inter-retinal fluid would flow through it into the vitreous and so make re-attachment possible. Lister considered that the presence of a hole made the outlook hopeless. The committee appointed by the Ophthalmological Society of the United Kingdom (1916) to consider detachment of the retina reported eighty-five cured detachments. Amongst these were three which showed a tear. Two of these were probably spontaneous cures. Thomson (1920) stated that it was useless to operate if a rent was present. Schreiber (1922) knew of only one detachment with a tear which had been cured. But Brons (1924) has described a detachment which re-attached after the tear healed spontaneously. He followed the healing process, observing that it commenced at the margins of the tear. Gonin (1924) has altered our outlook regarding the prognosis, if a tear exists. Six years ago he reported two cures, even though tears had been found near the ora serrata. Since then, in common with many others using his method, he has described many cures. He considers that the chances of success are less if the detachment has existed for more than three weeks. This is partly because the tear becomes increasingly difficult to find and because reapplication of the retina and the restoration of its function are hindered by degenerative changes (Gonin, 1930).

Dubois considers that the prognosis of traumatic detachments is generally favourable, but that if a tear is present, the outlook is not so good. He holds that when a tear has not resulted from traction on the retina of the vitreous, the prognosis is more favourable than when such a mechanism has produced the separation. The prognosis of detachments due to trauma is favourable if they are due to haemorrhage or oedema. If the tear is primary, that is, not due to the contraction of a cicatricial band, even though it be large as in an avulsion at the ora serrata, the outlook is good. When the tear is closed the detachment remains cured. But if the tear is due to a vitreous band, the detachment is active and the chance of cure remote (Dubois, 1929).

CHANCES OF RECOVERY. Schreiber (1920) reported 186 affected eyes, seen in the Heidelberg Clinic (1901–12), and claimed 7·5 per cent. of cures. Treatment consisted of rest, mercury, iodides, salicylates, subconjunctival injections, hot applications, and sweats. Only three of the fourteen patients operated on were cured. Seible (1916) reported 186 eyes and 6·5 per cent. cures. Only one was due to operation. 7·9 per cent. were improved. Uhthoff (1922) collected 351 re-attachments. Of these 24 per cent. followed operative treatment, 45 per cent. followed conservative treatment and 31 per cent. were spontaneous. Of his own patients, 9 per cent. finally re-attached. Fuchs (1923) quotes Leber's figures. 8·5 per cent. were cured as far as re-attachment is concerned, and 3·6 per cent. cured, if one means the restoration of moderately useful vision.

The report of the Ophthalmological Society of the United Kingdom in 1915 and 1916 is of interest. The standard of cure was re-attachment for at least six months, irrespective of proper function or visual result. In all eighty-five cures were reviewed, and of these fifty-one were in myopes. In forty-four cases, or just over 52 per cent., the result was attributed to some form of operative interference. In 28 per cent. the recovery was spontaneous, and in 20 per cent. such measures as rest and compressive bandaging were considered instrumental in producing the cure. In no case in which a tear was found did success follow operation, and in only three treated by other means is a cure mentioned. Darier (1920) reports his results from 1893 to 1913. The cases were treated by electrolysis, subretinal injection of iodine, and the intra-vitreous injection of air or saline. Sixty patients were treated, ten being cured, and twenty improved. After this date he altered his treatment, combining scleral puncture with sub-conjunctival hypertonic saline injections. Of forty-three cases, seven were cured and eleven improved. So in his combined series 16·5 per cent. were cured. Sourdille accepted as a standard of cure complete disappearance of the detachment, normal visual field and central acuity, which would enable the patient to read and to write. Amongst sixteen recent detachments he reported 62 per cent. cures over a period of at least six months. The vision in one was 10/10, but the majority were from 5/10 to 8/10. Amongst eighteen long-standing detachments no cures were reported, but 50 per cent. were improved. These results are a tribute to energy and perseverance. In some cases frequent punctures and injections were made. The only doubt one could have about these results would be the possibility of the inclusion of detachments due to pregnancy, and a large percentage of recent traumatic detachments. This is made probable by the fact that he reports no spontaneous cures. Deutschmann (1926), in a series of 539 retinal detachments, reported 177 cures, or just over 30 per cent. He treated forty-three by injection into the vitreous of the subretinal fluid, and the remainder by retinal puncture. These are unusually good records, and until recently, unique in the literature.

For contrast it is interesting to compare Vail's figures (1912). He sent a circular letter to 460 oculists. Of these 281 replied, and 250 had never treated a detachment successfully, though temporary improvement was reported to be common. Thirty-one oculists had cured forty-one detachments in all, four had two cures each, two had four cures each, and the remainder one each to their credit. One can exclude two of these cases as they occurred in pregnancy. In about one-half of the remaining thirty-nine, the cure, so Vail decided, was not convincing. He therefore concluded that the prospect of cure was less than 1 in 1000. This fortunately can be considered unduly pessimistic.

SIGNIFICANCE OF SITE, EXTENT AND DURATION. Though some oculists postpone operative measures until the detachment has reached the secondary stage and descended to the lower pole, it appears on *a priori* grounds that this is unwise. Not only does it mean that the detachment is older and therefore the vitality of the retina probably more affected, but also during the descent of the exudate irreparable damage may have been done to the central area of the retina. According to Sourdille, the most favourable site is the upper pole. This may be partly due to the fact that the majority of detachments commence in this area, and so a very considerable proportion of those found in the lower pole are secondary. The fact that they are then so far removed from the site of the initial lesion helps to explain why the chances of success are lessened. Detachments situated laterally are intermediate in prognosis, and the only ones with a worse outlook than the lower ones are those which are situated in the neighbourhood of the macula. These are difficult to approach by operation. In very extensive detachments it is this area that is most difficult to re-attach. So to a certain extent the variation of prognosis with site is dependent on the age of the separation. The outlook for a primary detachment at the lower pole is brighter than if it is secondary, other things being equal.

Complete detachments of course are almost hopeless. However, at times even those complicated by the presence of a cataract have been definitely helped by an extraction.

"It seems that two or three months represent the maximum limit, after which a detached retina can recover sufficient visual capacity for reading" (Sourdille). It is astonishing that such a delicate organ as the retina should remain for such a long time separated from its natural connections without degenerating completely. Cruise (1923) reported a remarkable case in which re-attachment occurred after ten or twelve years. Another detachment has been reported which re-attached spontaneously after three and a half years. In detachments of more than three months' duration functional cure is still possible. "It is less likely because, apart from the degeneration of the sensory cells, the retina loses its vital elasticity, and is incapable of unfolding. Degenerative changes appear in it and in the vitreous. As we have seen the early histologists considered these changes as primary" (Sourdille). Sourdille considered the detachments which bulge down in front of the disc easier to re-attach than the flatter detachments at the lower pole. This too may be due chiefly to the age of the separation.

SUMMARY. The outlook is considerably brighter than it was some years ago. In 1922, Terrien said that retinal detachment was then regarded as practically incurable. It is too soon finally to judge the permanence of Gonin's results, for the longest cure is of only three and a half years' duration. Few detachments that have adhered for this period have later re-detached. Paton's history of a recurrence after seventeen years is very exceptional. But when we remember the number of old and otherwise hopeless cases Gonin has successfully treated, we are justified in believing that it is by far the greatest improvement yet made in the therapy of this disorder.

Probably the prognosis of detachments due to a choroidal effusion is better than the others. The outlook in traumatic cases, according to Dubois, is generally favourable. Those detachments complicated by tears are certainly not hopeless, as they were until Gonin introduced his method of closing the opening. The prognosis in myopia, owing to the associated degeneration, is worse than it is in emmetropia and hypermetropia.

Gonin, Vogt and others, expert in the technique of ignipuncture, or rather expert in the all-essential finding and localising of the tear in the retina, have stated that the percentage of cures is approximately fifty.

It can be concluded that apart from those due directly to trauma and certain diseases, most "spontaneous" retinal detachments are secondary to some uveal disease. This disease may lead directly to effusion, and consequently a detachment, or indirectly, by producing degeneration in the vitreous, retina or ciliary body, may lead to a definite predisposition. With such conditions, a very slight trauma or transient vascular disturbance may be sufficient to precipitate the retinal separation, whether it be by means of a retinal tear, or a choroidal effusion. Because of the fundamental part played by uveal disease, it is necessary to go a step further back, for uveal disease is due to some morbid general phenomenon. Hence, much of the pathogenesis of retinal detachment will remain unsolved as long as so much in the field of general pathology is obscure.

REFERENCES

SPONTANEOUS RE-ATTACHMENTS

1874. HIRSCHBERG. *Klin. Beobach. aus der Augen. Wien*, 59.
1882. MOOREN. *Funf. Lustren. Ophth. Wirksamkeit.* **8**, 224.
1883. STILLING. *Arch. f. Augenheilk.* **12**, 332.
1883. SCHWEIGGER. *Ibid.* **12**, 52.
1891. HIRSCHBERG. *Zentralbl. f. p. Augenheilk.* **15**, 168.
1895. LEBER and FRANKEL, Z. *Zehender's Monatsbl.* **33**, 410.
1898. HORSTMANN. *Arch. f. Augenheilk.* **36**, 166.
1899. DE SCHWEINITZ, G. *Ophthal. Rev.* May, **18**, 150.
1907. REMAK. *Zentralbl. f. p. Augenheilk.* **31**, 262.
1916. FISHER, J. H. *Trans. Ophthal. Soc. U.K.* **36**, 396.
1919. CLAPP, C. A. *Amer. Jl. of Ophthal.* **2**, 474.
1921. SCHIÖTZ, I. *Klin. Monatsbl. f. Augenheilk.* Beilage, 67.
1923. BENEDICT and MUSSEY. *Amer. Jl. of Ophthal.* **6**, 286.
1923. GARDNER, M. C. *Med. Jl. of Australia*, **1**, 477.
1924. KRAUS. *Abst. Münch. med. Wochenschr.* March, 353.
1924. HILL, E. *Arch. of Ophthal.* **53**, 137.
1924. HIGHETT, H. C. *Brit. Jl. of Ophthal.* **8**, 226.
1927. SOUTER, W. C. *Brit. Med. Jl.* Discussion, Dec. 1127.
1928. NEAME, HUMPHREY. *Proc. Roy. Soc. Med.* Oct.
1929. FRY, W. E. *Arch. of Ophthal.* June, 745.
1929. HEINE, L. *Arch. f. Augenheilk.* **100–1**, 439.
1929. THOMSON, ERNEST. *Ophthalmoscope*, 7, 8.
1929. BIRCH-HIRSCHFELD. *Deut. med. Wochenschr.* **45**, 148.

THE EFFECT OF A RETINAL TEAR

1916. COMMITTEE. *Trans. Ophthal. Soc. U.K.* **36**, 352.
1920. THOMSON, E. S. *Arch. of Ophthal.* **49**, 563, 639.
1922. SCHREIBER, L. *Zeitschr. f. Augenheilk.* **48**, 171.
1924. BRONS. *Ibid.* **54**, 117.
1924. GONIN, JULES. *Zentralbl. f. p. Augenheilk.* 191.
1929. DUBOIS, H. *Ann. d'Ocul.* **166**, 81.
1930. GONIN, JULES. *Bruxelles-Méd.* 23rd March, 564.

THE CHANCES OF RECOVERY

1912. VAIL, D. T. *Trans. Amer. Acad. Ophthal. and Oto-Lar.* August.
1916. SEIBLE. *Klin. Monatsbl. f. Augenheilk.* **56**, 587.
1920. SCHREIBER, L. *Arch. f. Ophthal.* **103**, 750.
1920. DARIER, A. *Clin. Ophtal.* **24**, 10.
1922. UHTHOFF, W. *Deut. med. Wochenschr.* **48**, 115.
1923. FUCHS, E. *Text-book of Ophthal.* 7th edn., 593.
1926. DEUTSCHMANN. *Arch. f. Ophthal.* **117**, 146.

THE SIGNIFICANCE OF SITE, EXTENT, AND DURATION

1916. COMMITTEE. *Trans. Ophthal. Soc. U.K.* **36**, 359.
1923. SOURDILLE, G. *Arch. d'Ophtal.* **40**, 419.
1923. CRUISE, R. R. *Amer. Jl. of Ophthal.* **6**, 140.

SUMMARY

1923. PATON, L. *Amer. Jl. of Ophthal.* **6**, 140.

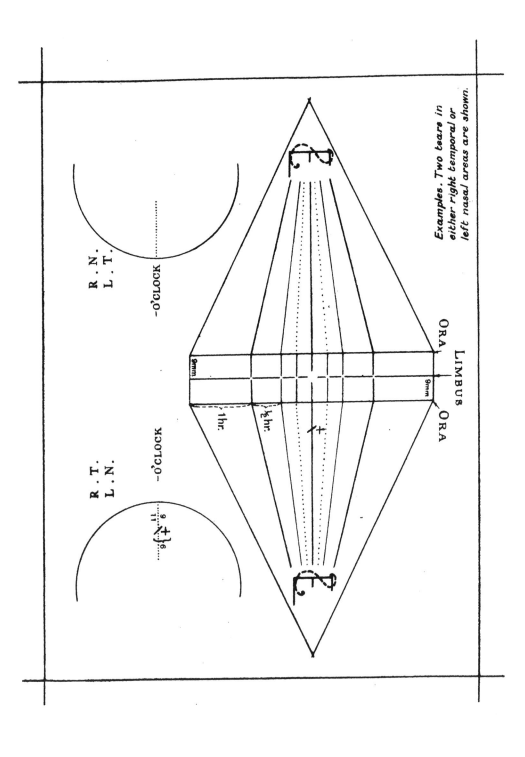

Examples. Two tears in either right temporal or left nasal areas are shown.

R . N.
L . T.

R . T.
L . N.

−O'CLOCK

−O'CLOCK

ORA

LIMBUS

ORA

9mm

9mm

1hr.

½hr.

APPENDIX

(a) METHOD OF USING CHART FOR PROJECTION OF RETINAL TEAR

Draw fundus details seen by indirect ophthalmoscopy in the semicircle marked *RT* or *LN*, etc., according to actual site of tear, viz. right temporal or left nasal quadrant, etc. The actual distances and sizes of tears must be given in D.D. (1·5 mm.) or in mm. The tear to be closed should lie on the meridian line which is marked "o'clock" and is dotted in mm. Reverse the chart so that the letters *E* (erect image) are erect. Fill in fundus details accurately above the semicircle so that the details lie at correct distances from the nearest vertical line, which represents the ora serrata. The tear to be closed must lie on or at a known distance from the horizontal line. This line will then represent the meridian (o'clock) of the tear.

Turn the chart over, hold it so that *S* is erect and towards the area of sclera overlying the tear. When the horizontal line is in the meridian of the tear, and when through the peep-sight one can see this line crossing the limbus, the fundus details will be in their correct position and their distances from the central line will represent their distances from the limbus.

(b) A FEW LANDMARKS ON THE TOPOGRAPHICAL ANATOMY OF THE SURFACE OF THE EYEBALL

There is danger of damaging the vessels, nerves, etc., during Gonin's operation.

The surface of the eyeball is divided into two halves. One-third of the anterior half is occupied by the cornea. Around the limbus of the cornea there is a circular zone, 5 to 6 mm. broad, underneath which lies the ciliary region. A circle drawn on the surface of the eyeball 8 mm. behind the limbus corresponds to the ora serrata. Another circle parallel to the limbus and from 13 to 14 mm. behind it, corresponds to the equator.

Most detachments occur between the ora serrata and the equator. Behind the equator are the four points of exit of the venae vorticosae—two above and two below. One must know their position.

The superior venae vorticosae are situated one on each side of the vertical meridian. The superior temporal vena vorticosa is 7 mm. behind the equator, while the superior nasal is 8 mm. behind the equator. The superior temporal is nearer the vertical meridian than the superior nasal.

The lower venae vorticosae are similarly arranged on the under surface behind the equator, one on each side of the vertical meridian. The inferior temporal vena vorticosa is nearer the vertical meridian and only 5 mm. behind the equator. The inferior nasal is further away and 6 mm. behind.

In other words, a band 3 mm. in breadth drawn around the eyeball from 5 to 8 mm. behind the equator, or from 18 to 21 mm. behind the limbus, will pass through the four points of exit of the four venae vorticosae.

The line of insertion on the eyeball of the superior oblique muscle lies between, and somewhat in front of the two superior venae vorticosae. It crosses the vertical meridian obliquely. Its temporal extremity is 14 mm., and its nasal extremity 19 mm. behind the limbus.

The ocular insertion of the inferior oblique is so far behind the equator that it is inaccessible by Gonin's procedure except at its temporo-anterior extremity, which is 18 mm. behind the limbus.

Finally, it is necessary to consider the position of the two long posterior ciliary arteries and nerves. They perforate the sclera, a nerve and an artery on each side of the optic nerve and run between the sclera and choroid in the horizontal meridian until they reach the ciliary region, where they distribute their branches to the iris, ciliary body, etc. Their course is underneath the recti externus and internus.

It must not be forgotten that all these figures are approximate only.

INDEX

www.ingramcontent.com/pod-product-compliance
Ingram Content Group UK Ltd.
Pitfield, Milton Keynes, MK11 3LW, UK
UKHW050116180125
453697UK00014B/445